MATHEMATICS AND
SEX

Clio Cresswell PhD, mathematician, writer, media presenter and educator, was born in England, had her childhood in Greece, was raised in the south of France, and attended university in Australia. Clio's somewhat unorthodox upbringing has greatly contributed to her varied and eclectic outlook on life. She enjoys all mental challenges and loves the extreme diversity of total body and intellectual workouts.

For several years a Visiting Fellow at the School of Mathematics, University of New South Wales, Clio is also a seasoned media performer. She features regularly on Australian television, radio and press.

MATHEMATICS AND
SEX

Clio Cresswell

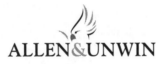

ALLEN&UNWIN

Allen & Unwin
83 Alexander Street
Crows Nest NSW 2065
Australia
Phone: (61 2) 8425 0100
Fax: (61 2) 9906 2218
Email: info@allenandunwin.com
Web: www.allenandunwin.com

National Library of Australia
Cataloguing-in-Publication entry:

Cresswell, Clio
   Mathematics and sex.

   Bibliography.
   ISBN 1 74114 159 1.

   1. Sex. 2. Sociology - Mathematical models. I. Title.

306.7

Set in 11/16 pt Bembo by Bookhouse, Sydney
Printed by Griffin Press, South Australia

10 9 8 7 6 5 4 3 2

CONTENTS

To Peter Herbert

ACKNOWLEDGMENTS

Meeting people you connect with intellectually is a rarity. Being able to develop ideas for a book with three has been a wonderful and privileged experience. Here are three fantastic people: Jo Paul and Colette Vella, the commissioning editor and senior editor from Allen & Unwin, and Peter Herbert, who is title-less and from nowhere in particular.

My life has also been blessed by dear friend Bruce Henry, who, with his emotional support and inquiring mind, contributes to all my projects well beyond the realm of colleague-to-colleague discussions.

My heartfelt thanks also goes to the School of Mathematics at the University of New South Wales for its constant support and encouragement. It has been an honour to be part of a community that truly embraces all kinds of innovative thinking.

I would like to especially thank a number of academics whose doors have always been open to me: Dr Peter Cooke, Associate Professor Jim Franklin, Dr David Nott, Associate Professor Norman Wildberger and Associate Professor Rob Womersley.

INTRODUCTION

For many people just seeing the words 'mathematics' and 'sex' in the same sentence is odd enough, let alone discovering there is a deep relationship between the two. But brace yourself because I'm about to awaken your senses to a new side of sex—and a new side of mathematics for that matter. Because believe it or not, sex is highly mathematical. Now I am not just talking about numbers and probabilities here. Sure, there is the arithmetic: the fabled 'thousand and one nights' of pleasure, the number of sexual partners, the number of times in a night, the frequency of orgasm, the quantity of sperm, and so on. Mathematics is certainly involved at this level. But the involvement goes much further. Mathematics is the study of patterns: their discovery, their interconnections and their implications. And in the context of sex, mathematics has uncovered a treasure-trove of sometimes unexpected but rich patterns and relationships.

Life is full of patterns and mathematics is uniquely suited to their discovery and explanation: from planetary motions, to fluctuations of the Dow Jones index, to human activities like walking, communicating, sleeping—or sex. With mathematics you can focus on the larger picture, you can zoom in to see the detail, and you can examine things from any angle. And sex affects us on so many levels it makes for a great topic in which to witness mathematics in action. There's love, the emotional side of sex, and there's partner searching, which we might call the pragmatic side of sex, and then there's orgasming, the physiological side, or, shall we say, the delightful side of sex. Mathematics uncovers aspects of all these areas that couldn't be uncovered otherwise. A plethora of sexual discoveries lies ahead.

But, let me backtrack a little. Mathematics—the study of patterns? How does that fit with the image of the bearded woolly-haired guy scribbling mathematical gobbledygook on a blackboard? Well, let's leave the 'bearded woolly-haired guy' cliché to one side for now. But the gobbledygook, well, if you can read it, has a voice. It tells us about patterns. The patterns form the centrepiece of mathematics, not the gobbledygook. And patterns, as pervasive as they are, lie at the heart of understanding life.

Sometimes mathematics is referred to as a language. And indeed it is. Patterns lend themselves to language-like representation. That's the gobbledygook on the blackboard. But language is not merely a collection of words, or symbols or gestures. Language is a means of communication. It is a vessel for conveying concepts. You can choose from a number of vessels. Poems capture things that can't quite be expressed in standard writing, and vice versa. Sometimes music or a song works better, sometimes a dance, a painting or a sculpture. Sometimes a performance artist will feel that hanging themselves on fishhooks from a beam is the only way they can express something deeply felt. This only goes to show how innate and important communication is to us.

We are driven to encapsulate the sensations we feel from our internal and external environments into language. We are constantly trying to convey ideas, to be heard and understood. But communication is also the central mechanism in place for us to make sense of things for ourselves. One of the best ways to learn something is to teach it to someone else. Through language, what might seem confusing, too complex and overwhelming can be elucidated. It is one of our most prized possessions. Whether it's Shakespeare, Madonna, or Renoir, something unique is being expressed. It is remarkable so many perspectives can be achieved through a finite set of words, grammar, notes and colours. Mathematics is another avenue of expression, helping us understand and convey phenomena we can't fully connect with otherwise. It is not the numbers or the symbols that are important; it is what is evoked through their combination. In the same way the steps make the dance and the colours make the painting, the symbols make the mathematics.

You will find such mathematical symbols and equations scattered throughout the book. Should this alarm you, let me put you at ease. They are not there to be understood. Their role is to create a strong link between their appearance and what they evoke. Showing translations of Ancient Egyptian hieroglyphics without the actual symbols just doesn't quite inspire the same awe. Mathematical symbols have the same aesthetic. Just think how $E = mc^2$ has captured people's imagination. Your mind is about to be charged with more. Having the equations there will also help debunk the idea that mathematics is some kind of weirdo ability to do elaborate calculations. Seeing equations in so many different and sometimes unexpected contexts is a way to develop a full appreciation for how mathematics really is so prevalent, fundamental and crucial.

Now of course, on top of bearded woolly-haired guys scribbling stuff, you could also be plagued by high-school mathematics nightmares of tedious times tables, formulae for areas of every single geometrical shape known to mankind and, if you are lucky, Farmer Joe's fence-length problems. In which case you might be feeling a bit out of touch with the use of mathematics as another creative avenue for you to express yourself. I tell you what though, it is much simpler than hanging yourself up for exhibition from a set of fishhooks!

Patterns and mathematics have always permeated our lives. Back in the days BC, around Egypt and Greece, rectangular fields were found to exhibit an amazing pattern: 'Hey did you know that every time you multiply the breadth by the length you get something called the area?' 'Wow!' came the reply. On opposite sides of the world, the Chinese and the Incas revelled in finding ways to tally up their harvests at breakneck speeds. While in India, using different methods to generate the most precise approximation of $\sqrt{2}$ ($= 1.41421356...$) was considered mesmerising.

Yes, fashions change. High-school mathematics may at times seem slightly stuck in that era, but there is a lot more. So let me jump to the 17th century when Isaac Newton, the Jean Paul

Gaultier of the mathematical scene, was born. He came along and introduced some pretty 'out there' ideas that mark a significant change in our culture. I don't know how Newton would feel about his ideas being compared to making pointy bras for Madonna, but you get my drift. Every now and then people come along who show us a completely new side of something with revolutionary effects.

Newton's favourite area of research was celestial mechanics: the hows and whys of planetary motion. Through his work he showed us the true power of equations. He used them to unearth a whole host of patterns never before seen. One of the best-known is how gravity is a property of objects that acts like a force. And with this relationship in mind, using equations again then led to why the planets in our solar system should follow the orbits they do. With ideas like these, Newton showed us there are some patterns in nature so intricate, so delicate, they can't be broken down into simpler ones, and that equations may be our only hope of capturing complex interactions. He also showed us the predictive power of mathematics, that mathematics is a way of foreseeing possible outcomes. And since Newton, using mathematics like this has become very popular. The big thing in the '80s, along with bubble skirts and boxing boots, was stock market prediction. Today, the big thing is mathematical biology. Well, that and having your jeans hang around your knees . . . Our bodies are teeming with patterns, and mathematicians have found themselves deluged by new patterns to play with. Molecules interweave to form strands of DNA, neurones fire in various sequences in the brain, and chemical reactions of all sorts interact. Mathematics is involved with them all.

Mathematics is forever growing, developing, and forging links with the real world, and this process draws on some amazing creative thinking. Give me any topic: engineering, law, sport—mathematics is in the scene doing just that. Oh yes, there is sex too of course. Sex comes into play powerfully in our lives and in so many ways. Sex can mean Calvin Klein can sell white T-shirts at almost any price. Isn't a white T-shirt a white T-shirt? No. A Calvin Klein label means sexy, sexy means sex, and we'll try all kinds of paths to reach that destination.

I have another tack. I propose casting fashion aside for a short while and using a bit of 'mathematical pattern-revealing' as another successful pathway to sex. By understanding some of the mathematical patterns underlying sexual behaviour, you'll be gaining access to some intriguing insights on the topic. And I know you want them. After all, we do live in a society where more than half the population read their horoscopes on a weekly basis, mostly in search of clues about their relationship issues (Chandhuri 2000; Mitchell & Tate 1998; Tyson 1982). Well, it is now time to indulge in some mathematical predictions. And let me be cheeky and suggest mathematics has a much, much, much better track record at forecasting events than astrology. So why hasn't the craze taken off? Well, some of the more powerful and therefore impressive research is very new. What you're about to see is some of the latest range of mathematical garments.

There could, of course, be a fear of being reduced to a series of equations. We live in an age bursting with one-stop chemical solutions to our human ailments and that can feel de-centering enough. Are you diabetic? Insulin will assist. Are you depressed? Serotonin enhancers may help. Can't stop thinking about that person you met last week? It could be that their pheromones initiated a chemical reaction in your brain. Are we just big chemical factories? What about love, devotion, loyalty? You can start to feel a bit ripped off. But when you become aware of the mathematics behind all that is going on with those chemicals you regain wonder in the human body. The works of Shakespeare were also written with mere words and rules of grammar, yet the way in which they are woven together expresses subtle phenomena of rare beauty. So too with the human body: chemicals interact with such style that the result is immensely elegant. Chemicals are just the alphabet in the underlying patterns of our behaviour, and mathematics shines light on these complex interactions. It doesn't change, tame, or constrain them. Mathematics is another way of experiencing things.

You may have dabbled in some sexual chemistry on your pathway to sex. Well, it's time to move further afield, it is time for some sexual mathematics.

Chapter 1

LOVE, SWEEEET LOVE

In the late '80s, a Harvard lecturer by the name of Steven Strogatz suggested an unusual class exercise to his students. The day's topic would be the Mathematics of Love. Professor Strogatz's motivations were plain cheeky. Confronted with the challenge of capturing his students' attention on the predictive powers of equations, he reworded a common undergraduate mathematics problem into a language he thought the students would relate to: the evolution of the love affair between Romeo and Juliet. His ingenuity should not be taken lightly: turning a group of hormone-raging twenty-year olds into utterly focused mathematical geniuses is a complex task. I wish I had been in his class to witness the full event.

Steven Strogatz didn't base his class exercise on extensive psychological research; he was just a Harvard lecturer having a bit of fun. But little did he realise he was actually beginning to make some mathematical sense of one of the great human emotions.

He presented the problem like this:

> Romeo is in love with Juliet, but in our version of the story, Juliet is a fickle lover. The more Romeo loves her, the more Juliet wants to run away and hide. But when Romeo gets discouraged and backs off, Juliet begins to find him strangely attractive. Romeo, on the other hand, tends to echo her: he warms up when she loves him, and grows cold when she hates him.

As you can see, emotions are a bit all over the place in this relationship. The question is, will they ever settle? What kind of relationship can Romeo and Juliet look forward to? The point of the exercise is to show how equations give insight into these real-life dilemmas. And no doubt many of the students related to the example.

The first step towards mathematical insight is to rewrite the terms of Romeo and Juliet's fickle affair mathematically. The translation is:

$$\frac{dR}{dt} = aJ, \frac{dJ}{dt} = -bR,$$

where R is for Romeo, and J for Juliet. How the letters are combined mimics how Romeo and Juliet find themselves interacting. For mathematicians, translating the problem into equations like this is natural. Mathematics is the study of patterns and this problem simply concerns behavioural patterns. Behavioural patterns are not static though and that's an important characteristic to bear in mind. Romeo's love depends on Juliet's responses and vice versa. Their interaction is fluid. It evolves. The pattern is forever changing and the equations above capture this too. The next step is to use mathematical techniques to analyse the equations, which will give answers about what kind of relationship can be expected.

As I touched on in the Introduction, being able to describe patterns of motion with mathematics originated in the 17th century with the work of Issac Newton. Now the study of evolving patterns forms a monumental part of mathematics. New discoveries in the area are being made around the world every day. And it's easy to see why: the stock market evolves; planes move over the Earth; the ozone layer changes shape. Mathematics enables you to find out how and why patterns change, whether the patterns are permanent or transitory, and whether other patterns can emerge. And the same techniques uncover what Romeo and Juliet can expect in their tempestuous relationship. The equations reveal a relationship characterised by a never-ending cycle of love and hate. Which doesn't sound all that appealing, but according to the mathematics, as they both cycle through these two emotions, they will reach simultaneous love one-quarter of the time. Not good enough? Or, maybe, not too bad? Do we usually achieve that much synchronicity with our loving relationships anyway?

The 'Romeo and Juliet' problem is rather straightforward, but the problem acts as a base from which we can study more complicated and realistic situations. And even small extensions to it yield some interesting findings. For example, here's Bart and Betsy's relationship:

Betsy's love is straightforward. It grows both with her attraction towards Bart as well as with his attraction towards her. But Bart has a commitment problem. His love only grows with Betsy's attraction towards him. It actually subsides when he feels his attraction to Betsy growing.

Will Bart's fear of commitment break the relationship? You can work through the mathematics and find it says 'no'. As long as Bart has some love for Betsy to begin with, if the couple stick to it they will eventually reach a state of ecstatic mutual love. Bart can resist all he wants, but he's going to feel that love whether he likes it or not! Now I know saying 'fear of commitment' can be like screaming 'fire': it is sure to grab attention. And while the true mathematics of commitment phobia might just be round the corner, we are still in the realm of oversimplified caricatures of relationships, with the ideas developed so far really still only serving to stimulate further analysis. Bart and Betsy's skeleton of a relationship might have a fairytale ending, but what about more realistic relationships? When do they share the same fate? What needs to be done to reach their mathematical understanding?

Well, not as much as you might first think. Have a look at the original 'Romeo and Juliet' problem again. Are you sure it doesn't ring any of the following bells?

★ You find yourself staring and staring into the depths of your partner's eyes, as if affected by a form of temporary paralysis.

★ You bore your friends to death talking about that one person all the time. You can't help it. It just makes you feel soooo gooood.

★ But are you ready for LIFELONG commitment?

★ Has a touch of self-doubt crept in for a millisecond?

★ Oh yes, yes, you must be ready. They're just so fantastic. You're once again walking around with that glowing tingling feeling.

★ Ooops, they feel down, your mood sinks with theirs.

★ Your heart aches with adrenaline and excitement.

★ You can't eat properly.

★ Hang on. Do you really have what it takes to fulfil all their dreams?

★ Do they?

★ Oh my god, not everything is going according to plan!

★ It never does!

Yep, love is often felt as a series of highs and lows. Love can be like riding an emotional roller coaster. Love can be like the game of emotional tug of war Romeo and Juliet experienced in Steven Strogatz's problem.

Our original mathematics is starting not to look so frivolous after all. And that is exactly what Italian mathematician Sergio Rinaldi realised. He began taking the mathematical study of romance seriously. Well, who best to study the rhythms of love but an Italian? And how better to start his study than with some of the most romantic poetry ever to be written: Petrarch's *Canzoniere*?

Proof in Petrarch

In the 14th century, an Italian poet Francis Petrarch wrote one of the most acclaimed collections of love poems of all time, *Canzoniere* ('Song Book'). *Canzoniere* consists of 366 poems (sonnets, songs, sestinas, ballads and madrigals), with more than

200 of them profiling Petrarch's passionate love for a married woman, Laura. Petrarch met Laura in the French city of Avignon at the age of twenty-three. From that point on, he spent twenty-one years writing about his attraction to her even though she never responded with similar feelings.

The poems are a classic account of the highs and lows so characteristic of passionate desire. Petrarch describes his delirious adoration of Laura, his despair over this unrequited love, his fantasies about a union, but also his impatience with Laura's coolness . . . then, amazingly, his absolute forgiveness of any negative feelings when she shows him the tiniest bit of attention. Laura's occasional glance or smile was enough to keep him so entranced, his passionate poetry continued for over ten years after her death—I guess glancing and smiling was quite hot stuff back then.

Was Petrarch a love-struck fool? Well, maybe, but he is considered the founder of Italian humanism. And his works are important markers in the transition from the Middle Ages to what we know as the modern era. *Canzoniere* in particular marks the birth of modern love-poetry. Petrarch captures the essence of human love with the tales of his character. Today, hundreds of years later, we are so accustomed to this idea of being love-struck, Harvard professors can use it as assumed knowledge on which to base a mathematics problem. Petrarch has been a great help, but he did leave us an intriguing problem. He didn't place the poems in *Canzoniere* in chronological order and most of them aren't dated. We are left with large gaps in our understanding of Petrarch's lyrical and psychological development. This puzzle has bugged scholars for centuries.

Now before I say more, let me awaken your senses with a little of his love poetry. The following quotations and English translantions appear in Sergio Rinaldi's 1998 article 'Laura and Petrarch: An intriguing case of cyclical love dynamics'. Look out for the signs of cyclical attraction.

From sonnet CCXXI:

Quale mio destin, qual forza o qual inganno
mi riconduce disarmato al campo
là 've sempre son vinto?
(What fate, what power or what insidiousness
still guides me back, disarmed, to that same field
wherein I'm always crushed?)

From sonnet LXXIX:

Così mancando vo di giorno in giorno,
sì chiusamente, ch'i' sol me ne accorgo
et quella che guardando il cor mi strugge.
(Therefore my strength is ebbing day by day,
which I alone can secretly survey,
and she whose very glance will scourge my heart.)

From sonnet LXIII:

Volgendo gli occhi al mio novo colore
che fa di morte rimembrar la gente,
pietà vi mosse; onde, benignamente
salutando, teneste in vita il core.

(Casting your eyes upon my pallor new,
which thoughts of death recalls to all mankind,
pity in you I've stirred; whence, by your kind
greetings, my heart to life's kept true.)

You can see by these three sonnets alone, Petrarch is riding your classic love-struck emotional roller coaster. I'm definitely feeling for the guy! Yet among all this heartache English psychologist Frederic Jones found the potential key to placing the undated poems. In 1995, he proposed a chronology for the poems based on the cyclical emotions of love. Frederic Jones first analysed the poems stylistically and linguistically. And then assuming Petrarch's emotions follow some continuity, he recreated their natural evolution and ordered the poems accordingly.

To do this he began by extracting the poems written while Laura was alive and grading them according to content. He gave negative marks for deep despair and positive ones for ecstatic love. So for example, the second extract above got a very bad mark. Then looking at the dated poems, about half of them, he saw a cyclical pattern become vaguely apparent in the grades. Petrarch seemed to revisit emotions about every four years. Frederic Jones placed the undated poems within the cycle by not only using their emotional content but also historical data about Petrarch's life, environment and travels. The dates seemed to work magnificently. But herein lies a false sense of security. This investigation involves a lot of subjective thinking. Frederic Jones could have been imagining full cyclical patterns where there just weren't meant to be any at all. Like when you can spot various animal figures in cliff faces or clouds.

The problem was screaming out for some mathematics. Frederic Jones saw that. And Italian Professor Sergio Rinaldi came to the rescue. Professor Rinaldi had a hunch *differential equations* might be able to sort this out. After all, Laura and Petrarch's emotional tangles were not too dissimilar to those of Steven Strogatz's Romeo and Juliet. They were just more realistic and therefore more complicated. By considering Laura and Petrarch's respective personality traits, he could use similar mathematics to forecast the development of their relationship and the dates of the poems. Just as Steven Strogatz unravelled Romeo and Juliet's emotional tangles mathematically, so did Sergio Rinaldi for Laura and Petrarch's:

$$\frac{dL}{dt} = -\alpha_1 L + \beta_1 \left[P \left(1 - \left(\frac{P}{\gamma} \right)^2 \right) + A_P \right],$$

$$\frac{dP}{dt} = -\alpha_2 P + \beta_2 L + \frac{\beta_2 A_L}{1 + \delta Z(t)},$$

$$\frac{dZ}{dt} = -\alpha_3 Z + \beta_3 P.$$

These three equations reflect the intertwined nature of Laura's interest, Petrarch's passion and his poetic creativity—one equation for each of these three critical influences of the *Canzoniere*. By the way, you probably guessed it but just in case you're wondering: the *L* stands for Laura, the *P* for Petrarch. The equations capture:

⋆ Laura and Petrarch's responses to the other's appeal.

⋆ The fading intensity of how they each feel for the other caused by lack of attention.

⋆ How Petrarch's love for Laura sustains his poetic inspiration.

⋆ How the more time Petrarch spends engrossed in his poetry the less time he spends indulging and therefore fostering his passionate obsession.

⋆ The fact that Laura is a beautiful high-society lady who naturally attracts flirtations and that she quite likes Petrarch's attention to a degree.

⋆ Laura's sensitivity to Petrarch's advances.

⋆ Laura's disdain for Petrarch should he place too much pressure on her: sometimes his poetry becomes quite intense, sometimes to her embarrassment it was sung in public.

⋆ The subsiding of Laura's antagonistic feelings over time; after all she is flattered by Petrarch's attention.

⋆ How Laura feels sorry for Petrarch when his poetry shows signs of too much desperation and therefore how she returns to flirting with him.

⋆ The fact that, like most people, Petrarch loves to be loved and hates to be hated.

All that is in those three measly little equations . . . now you can't tell me the mathematics doesn't look simpler than all of that! Believe it or not the last emotional response 'one loves to be loved and hates to be hated' is encapsulated quite elegantly by $\beta_2 L$ in the second equation.

With mathematical training, those three equations can be understood quite readily. They work together to describe the intricacy of the situation and the resulting behaviour, if any, of this messy emotional web. Sergio Rinaldi analysed the equations and found that, sure enough, Petrarch was doomed to relive his emotional highs and lows and that a four-year cycle can emerge effortlessly. The mathematics shows the cyclical pattern is part of the parcel. With such evidence of repeated emotional waves, today Petrarch would probably be put on Prozac. Sergio Rinaldi's mathematical evidence beautifully complements Frederic Jones's findings. Frederic Jones now has mathematics to back him up on his placement of the undated poems. If his placement was a fiction of his imagination, it is to be commended!

With such a resounding success on his hands, how could the Italian not pursue further equations of love?

More Rinaldi love

OK, so some of us have experienced love's emotional roller coaster, but few of us have endured it for twenty-one years like Petrarch! If a relationship lasts, feelings more than likely stabilise; beautiful emotions associated with security, respect and deep friendship emerge. But don't worry if that seems a bit picture perfect. I don't think we're meant to be feeling the love–serenity thing 24/7, and of course what 'it' is, is not cast in stone. Oh dear, here we go again: 'What is the definition of love?' Yawn. We've all heard this so many times we're likely to pass out from boredom before the question is fully posed. And guess what? There is still no right or wrong answer. If you have ever wondered if what you are feeling is really love, don't beat yourself up, so has a huge scientific community. And they have been working exclusively on the concept for years. And still will be in many years to come. What does characterise the evolution of throws of passion into deep, emotional, long-lasting bonding? How long does it take? Does one always follow the other? Behavioural psychologists, evolutionary psychologists, cultural anthropologists, psychoanalysts, sociologists, they've all had a go at answering.

For example, Elaine Hatfield, a professor of psychology at the University of Hawaii, and her collaborators over the years, see deep affection or 'companionate love' as they call it, as a most definite follow-on from passionate love. Robert Sternberg, a professor of psychology at Yale University, is famous for his triangular theory. For him love results from the interaction of passion, commitment and intimacy, each of which follows its own course in a relationship. Psychologists Phillip Shaver and Cindy Hazan put more of an evolutionary spin on things. They believe love is an integration of attachment, care-giving and sexual behaviours. Attachment is seen as an extension of that first emotional bond we feel as infants towards our primary caregivers. The three behaviours are thought to come into play at various levels as love develops. Attachment theory is big at the moment.

Now, with Sergio Rinaldi, mathematicians are having their say on the theory of love as well. Equations had so successfully captured the romance between Strogatz's version of Romeo and Juliet, and that between Laura and Petrarch, that Sergio Rinaldi decided to take these as models on which to build equations that would reflect the emotional ties found in your more average everyday relationships. The equations of love he developed look like this:

$$\dot{x}_1(t) = -\alpha_1 x_1(t) + R_1(x_2(t)) + I_1(A_2),$$
$$\dot{x}_2(t) = -\alpha_2 x_2(t) + R_2(x_1(t)) + I_2(A_1).$$

Two lines for what can drive us so insane? Seems a bit scary. The R doesn't stand for Romeo and there is no J for Juliet, nor L for Laura. Instead the two lovers remain known as lover number 1 and lover number 2, and the amount of love one feels for the other as x_1 or x_2 (depending on who's feeling the love). Really, it can't get sexier than that, can it? Well maybe Rinaldi isn't the completely passionate Italian but believe me, if you want to understand love, it's all in there:

★ How appealing one lover finds the other. This could be physically, intellectually, financially, socially, whatever tickles their fancy.
★ How we love to be loved and hate to be hated. Yes, this goes for most of us, not just Petrarch. It has been tested and tested. As any introductory social psychology book will tell you, your average person will feel more love for someone if they sense their feelings are being reciprocated.
★ How our interest in the other can fade sometimes for reasons not associated with how sexy they are or how much they care about you. The extreme case being after a break-up, when in time, your feelings for the other die out. (These calculations exclude various forms of psychoses, such as stalking, where this does not happen.)

Now you may be thinking, surely there's more to love than this. How about the number of times I've had my heart broken?

Or, what if I'm really going for a promotion at work and am not receptive to companionship? Or, wouldn't I weigh things completely differently if children from previous relationships were involved? Well, yes, these things do come into play, but they are extras, things that are very dependent on specific situations. Adding them into the mix would be heading back towards specific case studies, like those of Romeo and Juliet and Bart and Betsy. Sergio Rinaldi concentrated on identifying the essential ingredients for love.

Once the equations are analysed, they predict the fate of two people affected by the above bare minimum of emotions. Sergio Rinaldi was interested in uncovering the development of a couple's emotions right from their very first encounter. His ground rules: two people meet, and having never set eyes on each other before, feel completely indifferent towards each other. What can happen? Well, pages of calculations, diagrams, and theorems later, one of his first findings was this: if they are attracted to each other, they can fall in love. Anticlimax? Not at all, it shows he's on the right track. And what the equations also suggest is how the love is affected. Feeling like your relationship has lost a bit of oomph? Well the famous *law of comparative dynamics* and the *theorem of maximum relative variation* have a word or two for you.

First, Rinaldi's equations tell us that all it takes for both individuals' love for each other to be boosted is for one person in the relationship to increase their appeal: they could shave their legs or chest, or other parts; they could buy a sexy top; or suddenly make a lot of money. It could be almost anything. What is good to know, though, is it is the partner's love that will be most affected. A small investment in appeal can lead to a large return in love. If you are worried about how love grows, you've got to like that.

Second, if one person becomes more responsive to the other's lovey-dovey feelings, then again this will boost both individuals' love for each other. Sometimes we feel more mushy than at other times. This might be when we love to be loved more. Here, it is the person who has increased their sensitivity that will actually be most affected. But importantly, both will love more—you've got to like that also.

And lastly, there appears to be a clear distinction between two different types of couples. Couples always able to recover from any temporary negative influences on their relationship, and couples either able to recover but equally able to see their feelings for each other completely deteriorate. Rinaldi calls these robust and fragile couples. Remember Bart and Betsy? Their relationship was tinted with Bart's fear of commitment but they survived, they were robust. The description of their interactions might have been threadbare but with added sophistication we recover similar patterns. However this is where the mathematics becomes awfully tantalising because how to find out which class your relationship fits into, is a question still waiting for an answer.

But, what Rinaldi's mathematics reveals all rings true. And while his equations are a somewhat crude simplification of reality, the fact that they do ring true only highlights their beauty. Sergio Rinaldi has begun to isolate what makes love tick. The next step is for psychologists to use his findings for their studies. And with their findings, the equations can be further refined to find out more. And so the process continues with the questions of love becoming easier to ask and answer.

Rinaldi on love gone bad

Part of Sergio Rinaldi's role is, therefore, to grab psychologists' attention. And finding out when healthy couples can have healthier relationships might not exactly be the best way to do that. Sergio Rinaldi, working with another Italian mathematician Alessandra Gragnani, and an Austrian mathematician, Gustav Feichtinger, turned this field of mathematics towards the study of neuroses. Their goal was to find out if accounting for certain neuroses in the love equations would then lead to the mathematical prediction of a tempestuous relationship. Remember the toing-and-froing in Laura and Petrarch's relationship? All twenty-one years of it, even beyond her death. What types of couples can expect such a crazy never-ending cycle of emotional ups and downs?

Rinaldi's initial focus: *security*.

Clear differences have been found in the way *secure* versus *non-secure* people respond to attachment. Canadian psychologists Dale Griffin and Kim Bartholomew have written extensively on the topic. A secure person has a general positive outlook about themselves and others, a good dose of self-esteem, and is comfortable with intimacy. A secure person responds positively to feeling attracted to someone and to relationships. Non-secure people also respond positively to attachment because they aren't complete fruit loops . . . but their positive feelings last only up to a certain point. Once their limit is reached they can start to respond quite negatively. A non-secure person becomes anxious at the idea of becoming too close to someone. Can you see the pattern? Secure people feel increasingly positive about their involvements, while non-secure people feel increasingly positive at first but then experience a drop. It is a pattern begging to be described with mathematics.

But after doing just that, Sergio Rinaldi and his co-workers found it wasn't enough. Adding the possibility of an eventual freak-out by a non-secure person didn't mean the relationship was going to become an emotional yo-yo. Not to worry, fully aware most of us carry more than one glitch in our personalities, the trio built in another possible neurosis to their equations.

Their focus this time: *synergism.*

Synergism is a curious phenomenon. Ever noticed how mothers tend to have a biased view about how attractive or smart their children are? Or maybe how lovers have similar biases towards each other? That's what Sergio Rinaldi calls synergism: our tendency to have an overly positive opinion about the attributes and abilities of the people we care for. In one of Jeffry Simpson, Steven Gangestad and Margaret Lerma's experiments, performed at Texas A&M University where Jeffry Simpson was residing, the men in relationships scored a bunch of unknown women as being, on average, 10 per cent less attractive than the group of single men did. It is as if nature issues us with special sexy-goggles when entering a relationship. This could be its way of helping us stay in one so we can pass on our genes more successfully. So if your boyfriend is forever telling you your ass looks hot, he's probably not pacifying you at all, OK? He truly is just reporting what he sees!

Sergio Rinaldi describes the synergic pattern as follows. The more love you feel for someone the more attractive you will find them, and so the more you will love to be loved by them. There's a feedback loop happening there. Bingo! This is where tempestuous relationships pop up. Depending on whom you pair up with, you could be in for some serious emotional yo-yoing. If you and your lover are both secure, then it doesn't matter how synergic or not either of you might be, your relationship is predicted to remain pretty stable. However, if one of you is secure but highly synergic—highly sensitive to the other's love and looks—and the other is non-secure but not synergic at all, then you have excellent mathematical cause to expect there to be a cyclical emotional pattern just around the corner. But all is not lost if you are cyclically destined. Security and synergism can and do vary. They can be moderated, and changes can enable a couple to reach peaceful gaga bliss. By working on your security and synergism traits, you might see your relationship transform in one of the following ways: either the cycles in your relationship could simply fade away or otherwise they could become interrupted by bursts of warm fuzzy love that lessen in frequency until everything settles. Either way, the roller coaster ride ends.

We now have a mathematical explanation of why the initial turmoil associated with falling in love may fade: insecurity and synergism become less pronounced.

This is becoming sickly sweet, I know, but let me finish with another small extension Sergio Rinaldi made to his love equations. Perhaps in a moment of universal compassion, Rinaldi took a step back, and looked at the larger picture, wondering if his love equations could contribute anything at the community level.

On the community scale, large numbers of couples are interacting at any one time and one person's appeal not only affects their partner but also affects a number of people around them. Increasing one's sex appeal not only increases our partner's desires but also that of others. Surely this cause for temptation leads to community unrest. Could varying sex appeal levels in a community cause love wars to explode?

By finding what patterns emerge from a whole host of love equations in action concurrently, Sergio Rinaldi found only one guarantee for a content community: everyone has to be paired up with a partner of similar appeal. As if there was some kind of sex appeal ranking and no one had made a mistake and everyone was in a relationship with someone of the same ranking.

Is this earth-shattering news? Surely this kind of hierarchy would be forced on us naturally, if we all aim to pick our best option possible when it comes to lifelong companionship. And a whole bunch of research does show a tendency for people to pair off according to similar levels of sex appeal (Berscheid et al. 1971; Zajonc et al. 1987). Could utter community contentment be just around the corner? How lovely. But does community contentment mean anything about how we feel individually? I'll return to this in Chapter 5 because our fight for our best possible partner creates interesting patterns in contentment levels.

$$\partial x \mathop{/} \partial x + \partial x \mathop{/} \partial x + \partial x \mathop{/} \partial x + \partial x \mathop{/} \partial x + \partial x \mathop{/} \partial x + \partial x \mathop{/} \partial x + \partial x \mathop{/} \partial x$$

Initially, when we fall for someone we feel giddy, uplifted and hyper-alert. We're on a love high. But the slightest influence can send our emotions soaring in the other direction. We experience cravings for love, we crash dramatically following a break-up, and we feel the intensity of the rush decrease as time goes on. No wonder love has been studied in the context of addiction. Professors Andreas Bartels and Semir Zeki of University College,

London, found areas of the brain activated by the use of cocaine also became active when lovers were shown photos of their sweethearts. And a number of studies have shown people in love have high blood levels of PEA (phenylethylamine), a natural amphetamine found in chocolate.

Could love actually be unhealthy? Maybe it is like red wine, it is good for you as long as it is in moderation. And here is where a problem may lie ahead. Stanton Peele, a New York psychotherapist, warns we are staring straight down the barrel at a society of addicted love freaks. Western culture appears to have gone berserk over passionate love. From movies, to books, to the lives of superstars we want to emulate, we are bombarded with the ideal of two becoming one. Many of us expect romantic dinners and hand-in-hand walks on a beach with someone we find intellectually and physically stimulating, who is our best friend, with whom we have great sex, and with whom we share a sense of humour and seek similar fun. Some people even add 'good provider' to this list!

Reaching this goal is also seen as a major achievement, so we pursue it like hound dogs on scent. But it hasn't always been this way and still isn't in many places around the world. Love has often been secondary to family, marriage and economic realities. Helen Fisher of Rutgers University has noted the Tiv people of Africa might feel the passion we call 'love' but it seems in their language they call it 'madness'.

We need to understand more about love. And something we can't even define properly yet is sure to be bursting with some of the most complex and amazing patterns. Cycles of emotional ups and downs are but one pattern. The possibilities abound. Some patterns will be so unfathomable there will be no hope of finding them without mathematics. I urge you to keep your eyes and mind open.

Have certain types of lovers made you feel more insecure than others? Were the initial throws of passion more intense in those relationships? Does alcohol make you more love friendly or love adverse? When does lack of sex start influencing your judgment on potential soul mates? How long does it take for you to unwind after work and be ready for some schmooping up with your lover? Maybe a particular type of music helps?

Have I got your mind ticking over? I'll have you thinking like a mathematician in no time at all!

Chapter 2

MARRIAGE AND
THE HAPPILY EVER AFTER

So you're in love. You've reached the end of the emotional roller coaster ride of passion. Now the two of you feel a strong sense of intimacy and companionship. You never knew emotions could go so deep. You feel ready to marry. Wait! Are you really ready? Aren't we bombarded with headlines reminding us that a large percentage of marriages end in divorce? In a recent report, the US Census Bureau estimates a 50 per cent rate for first marriages (Krieder & Fields 2001). Let me say that again: 50 per cent! And the rate traditionally goes up for second marriages! Forget about passion and depth of feelings, how can anyone ever be ready to marry in the face of that sort of statistic?

Well, this is one time where most of us choose to be the optimist and see ourselves as part of the percentage that won't divorce. The numbers don't scare us. Instead, we choose to see them as reminders that we should pick our partners carefully and, perhaps more than anything else, that relationships are hard work. What we need to focus on then is how to work towards a long-lasting fulfilling relationship. We need to learn some tricks that will ensure the marriage lasts. Is it about accepting your partner for who they are? Are all the myths about the long-term decay of that lustful feeling true? Should we forget the passion and focus on companionship?

I think I can safely say you haven't considered picking up a mathematics textbook when thinking about such questions. *Men Are From Mars, Women Are From Venus* by John Gray maybe? Something else? There are literally thousands of books to choose from. Not so long ago, in the 1970s, you more than likely would have turned to the book, *Fascinating Womanhood* by the popular author Helen Andelin. She suggested women should be waiting at the door with a cold martini in hand when their husbands come home from work—not drinking the martini, but offering it. And, as a thank you, the husband was advised to buy his wife a new white good like a stove or fridge.

Now you can still try this approach to attaining unbounded happiness in marriage, but I think I can persuade you that a couple of mathematical techniques might have a better rate of success.

Hold it in or say it out loud?

We've all been in a situation where someone is getting on our nerves but for various reasons we hold our emotions in and behave quite politely: at work, while driving, grocery shopping... Now I think about it, don't we spend most of our day holding in those emotions?

However, work issues we can leave at work (ideally), and other drivers and shoppers we will never see again, but what if our partner is the someone doing the something sending us slowly but surely INSANE! They could be totally unaware of what they are doing and it may mean nothing to them to stop. Should we let them know? But then they might feel hurt and this could cause ripples in the relationship. So it might be better not to say anything and simply focus on understanding why they are doing it. Then again, if we take this approach, we might feel like we are compromising too much and so start feeling edgy about the relationship. Confused? What is the best approach if you want to safeguard your relationship? Should we be brutally honest or empathetic?

Until recently it has been thought empathy was the way to go. Dysfunctional marriages were thought to arise when partners' expectations for the marriage were too high. Marriage therapy focused on cultivating an 'x-ray vision' in which partners were able to see the lifetime wounds underlying any of the other's hostile behaviour (Hendrix 1990, p. 76). Countless couples have been told they need to really get to know their partner, and embrace all their strengths as well as weaknesses. They need to fully understand and accept who they are and what they do, and become a true team. Sounds fantastic. But come on, doesn't that also sound a little saintly? Can any human really aspire to being that angelic? Surely, asking us to intellectualise our emotions to that degree sounds suspicious!

It has been questioned. For example, in his 1993 book *Couples Therapy: A Non-traditional Approach*, marriage therapist Daniel Wile does discuss how partners may need to stop 'compulsively compromising' and develop 'an ability to complain'. So, again, what should we do, more sympathising or more whining? We can't just chop and change between approaches to marriage therapy casually, the cost of potentially stuffing up a whole set of marriages in the process is too high. Clearly, there is a need to test the theories—and without using human guinea pigs. How? With mathematics, of course! And psychologists, John Gottman and Catherine Swanson, and mathematician, James Murray, all from the University of Washington have done just that.

Professor John Gottman is a bit of a guru in the area of marriage. By examining partners' heart rates, facial expressions, and how they talk about their relationship to each other and to other people, he claims more than 90 per cent accuracy in predicting break-ups. John Gottman has published an abundant amount of academic articles and books, and won numerous awards. He and his wife Julie have even set up the Gottman Institute to provide hands-on marital help to couples and all sorts of health-care providers. At the University of Washington he founded the Family Research Laboratory where for years couples have subjected themselves to a host of experiences for his studies: from psychological tests, to skin conductivity measurements, to being videotaped interacting for twelve hours in their fake laboratory apartment. By the way, his original degree was a Bachelor of Science with majors in mathematics and physics.

As part of his studies John Gottman has come up with the Specific Affects Coding System. Sounds terribly important, doesn't it? We'll call it SPAFF. SPAFF is a code that weighs up and scores positive and negative interactions during a couple's conversation. For example, anger, sadness and whining score negatively, while humour, interest and joy score positively. The categorisation is done according to the content of what partners say and the context in which they say it, as well as their tone, facial expressions, and their gestures. No stone is left unturned. Each partner receives a series of scores for a conversation, one for each turn they have at speaking. When couples are discussing an issue they disagree about in their relationship, like money, in-laws or sex, the average is an utterance or a score every six seconds. Now if you decide to go and measure how long one of your utterences lasts for in a conversation with your partner, please note to discard any of the superfluous 'uh huhs', 'yeahs' and 'mm-humms' scattered throughout the conversation. They don't count in SPAFF scores. Although, I'm sure they do count in the following categories: footballers giving interviews, rappers expressing their innermost feelings, and any conversation with Billie Bob Thornton.

SPAFF and similar codes have been John Gottman's tools of success. He has gathered innumerable amounts of data on couples' attitudes and feelings, and has uncovered key components in couples' interactions that point to marriage stability or, alternatively, divorce. He has got it down to such a fine art, all he needs to make an assessment is for a couple to be videotaped torso up for fifteen minutes. Yet after focusing on data gathering and statistical analysis for years, John Gottman and his colleagues realised that while such methods were a great way to uncover *relationships* between different aspects of a partnership, they would need to turn to some 'hard-core' mathematical equations to uncover possible *mechanisms driving these relationships*. Their point is that getting a grip on the mechanisms underlying marriage is what will lead to a true understanding of how marriage works. And so these mechanisms will more than likely also reveal new methods to help couples live or build conjugal bliss.

This is what led John Gottman, Catherine Swanson, and James Murray, to encapsulate fifteen minutes worth of newlywed SPAFF scores into:

$$W_{t+1} = a + r_1 W_t + I_{HW}(H_t),$$
$$H_{t+1} = b + r_2 H_t + I_{WH}(W_t).$$

As couples discuss a source of disagreement around 150 scores are gathered. As I said earlier, about one score every six seconds: one to the husband, one to the wife, one to the husband, one to the wife, and so on. The equations actually show how one score follows another. They get tailored specifically to each spouse according to their general mood at the time of the conversation, their everyday temperament, their mood fluctuations when they deal with all kinds of problems, and—this is the crucial part—how their partner influences their mood. That's the *influence function* represented by the letter *I*! And that's exactly what John Gottman and his colleagues were investigating. How do spouse's moods change according to what the other says? If one spouse is interacting with a positive attitude but the other with a negative one, how long is it before both spouses end up feeling negative?

This is where the concept of a 'negativity threshold' comes in. Both partners possess this threshold, which, when crossed, means they will become negative or express their discontent. Until they reach this point, however, they will remain positive or empathise.

A negativity threshold might be suggested intuitively if you observe couples interacting long enough, but whether it exists or not is another matter. I mean, what is it exactly? How can a value be associated to it? Ascertaining if someone feels good about something is one thing and seems easy enough, but pinpointing when positive feelings turn negative is something else. Negativity thresholds need to be calculated using SPAFF scores and the above equations. This is our only way to get an initial grasp of this innovative concept.

So that is exactly what John Gottman and his colleagues did. Over a hundred newlywed couples underwent analysis so negativity thresholds could be found. And sure enough, six years later, a link emerged between negativity thresholds and stable marriages. But which couples survived the best? Was it those whose partners had low negativity thresholds? Where whinging happened sooner than later? Or was it those whose partners had high negativity thresholds? That is, where individuals empathised for as long as they could? Believe it or not, marriages where there was whinging definitely came out on top! Actually, the whinging came mostly from the wives. However the final recommendation by Gottman's team of mathematical psychologists was, whether you are husband or wife, 'Don't let things ride and have a chance to build up.' We have a mathematically tested secret to a long marriage: Low tolerance = long-term happiness.

So couples who continually repair their relationship end up feeling the most positive about their marriage. It appears high standards are good because they work as goals couples can reach for. This may seem counterintuitive. You might think that if your marriage is in a constant state of repair then maybe it is seriously flawed, or that high standards associated with the willingness to whinge would be more overwhelming than helpful—but not so.

Now predicting which couples are going to end up happy and which ones are not is one thing. Perhaps more importantly, the mathematical isolation of the 'negativity threshold' has great potential when it comes to saving relationships. Could our high divorce rates be related to most couples having too high a threshold? As John Gottman and his colleagues point out, it has been found couples wait on average six years from when they sense a serious problem in their marriage before they seek professional help. Now that may be because seeing a marriage shrink can feel scary—not to mention be quite expensive—but it may also be because of people's high thresholds. Especially since the couples that do end up on a shrink's couch usually find themselves relapsing into unhappiness after one to two years. Could marriage therapy be improved if it focused on resetting a couple's thresholds lower? Marriage therapy successfully deals with current issues but it could be failing at installing lifelong skills to prevent relapses.

Needless to say, sustaining a happy and stable marriage involves more than not compromising. But if things haven't been going so well in your marriage, it might be a good idea to first ask your partner: 'Honey, have you been letting your marital negativity threshold rise again? I know I have and I for one am not going to take it anymore!' And for single people out there, if you do ever feel the urge to plunge into a relationship, remember to establish a low negativity threshold right from the first date. And then if things reach the stage of marriage, I'd suggest a little bit of a word modification at the ceremony: 'I promise to love, honour and cherish you always . . . but I draw the line at your mother, I want you to take driving lessons, and as for your bathroom habits . . . ' Let me know how the marriage turns out.

Polarisation

So here is my next piece of mathematical marital advice. Be aware of polarisation. I know that sounds like something that would happen to your car battery, but as it turns out it's something that could happen to you. Do any of the following situations sound familiar? Jennifer wants to spend a large wad of money on the garden but her husband Brad thinks it would be wasteful; Brad and Jennifer don't see eye to eye on politics, so when it's time to vote they end up in a heated debate; Brad always ends up taking the garbage out, Jennifer never does. When people find themselves with extreme opposite points of view or behaving in diametrically opposite ways, we have polarisation.

You might think polarisation is simply part of the human condition, that it would be foolish to expect us to agree on everything. But with eight pages of mathematics Adam Kalai from Carnegie Mellon University and Ehud Kalai from Northwestern University found a surprising origin for this state of affairs.

For insight, let's return to our exemplar couple: Brad and Jennifer. Brad and Jennifer like to donate to charities every year. But Jennifer is a tiny bit more generous than Brad. She would like to see 10 per cent of their combined income go to charities while Brad would like to stop at 8 per cent. Because they are the perfect couple, they discuss the issue over dinner one night and decide on a compromise: over the year Jennifer will allow herself to donate 5 per cent of their combined earnings to charities and Brad will allow himself to donate 4 per cent; the end result being 9 per cent of their combined income going to charities. Do they live happily ever after?

Not necessarily. Here's what's likely to happen. Brad really doesn't want that extra per cent of their income to go. So the next year he decides to donate a smidgin less, thinking it compensates a little for Jennifer's excesses. And it won't really matter in the bigger scheme of things anyway. Jennifer in turn decides to give a smidgin more. Her rationalisation is the same as Brad's. And the year after, the same thing happens: Brad donates a little bit less and Jennifer a little bit more. Each is overcompensating for the other's perceived bias. And before you know it, a few years later, Brad is donating zilch while Jennifer is donating the full 10 per cent. Bingo! We have polarisation and the perfect scenario for a huge argument. Which, as you notice, happens even though Brad and Jennifer started off with similar views on charity donation. Insert more of these situations into a relationship and it's going to become a pretty miserable one. And while charity donation is not part of everyone's life portfolio, there are plenty of other situations. Think bathroom cleaning. Isn't it always the case the 'cleaner one' ends up cleaning for two? Think disciplining children. Doesn't one parent invariably end up known as a tyrant and the other a pushover? Could couples be feeling worlds apart in a whole number of areas where the true disagreement is in fact minute?

Here is where mathematics steps in. How small is minute? And what characterises agreement? Maybe as long as the shower has no mould growing on it and the mirror is devoid of toothpaste splatters, you will both deem the bathroom to be clean. Now if one of you decides to dust each shelf in the cosmetics cabinet, that's a bonus, but overall it's not going to add much to how satisfied you are with the cleaning. Mathematicians can get on top of such detail. They have ways to consider the worth of events to people. Ways based on a formula called a *utility function*. With it, mathematicians place values on worth in a whole variety of fashions. For example, if a job can be broken up into a number of smaller ones, the *utility function* might serve to simply sum up the worth of each of these. You might have:

$$shower\ cleaned\ +\ mirror\ wiped\ +\ cosmetic\ cabinet\ dusted\ =\ clean$$

where a clean shower scores between 0 and 10, a clean mirror between 0 and 5, and a clean cosmetic cabinet between 0 and 1. The shower is the most important item to clean and so doing so is worth more.

But this is just one of many others; another approach might be for the *utility function* to change the worth of each of the smaller jobs depending on how they were completed the time before. Was the cosmetic cabinet cleaned last time? Maybe we can carry over its score for a few more cleans. And you can go on like this, coming up with a whole load of ways to take account of worth.

Is this sounding obsessive or what? Well, such detail can actually reveal a lot about a situation. And this is how Adam Kalai and Ehud Kalai proved the *polarisation lemma*, the title given to their small piece of mathematics that basically says the following: if you assign worth to an event by simply breaking it up into smaller events and adding up your appraisal of each (as in my first bathroom cleaning example), then watch out because as parties aim to maximise their worth, polarisation becomes inevitable—the tiniest difference in opinion (worth) will create a huge drift in outcomes down the track.

The polarisation lemma spells bad news, that's true. But there is a way out. Become aware you are heading down that path, and avoid it. Remember, KNOWLEDGE IS POWER.

First point to remember is how such situations occur even though the two parties begin with quite similar views. You and your partner might feel you have become like two head-butting antelopes over some issue when really that couldn't be further from the truth. Once you've isolated that, and maybe had a good laugh, here is my mathematician's advice. Toss a coin!

You see the idea is to change your strategy vis-à-vis the problem so as to avoid the continual tug in opposite directions. If you toss a coin, and make the loser clean the bathroom, you introduce some randomness into the problem. Sticking to this strategy will mean both people will get to clean the bathroom and to their own level of satisfaction. There will be that small discrepancy, but at least it won't end up blowing out of proportion. It is even easier to understand in the context of charity donation. If Brad and Jennifer toss a coin each year and the winner chooses how much of their combined income goes to charities, then some years they will donate 10 per cent and some years 8 per cent. The average will be 9 per cent and the issue should never be brought up again.

Tossing a coin is a way to force the other person to accept your small deviations from their beliefs. And the blame gets laid on chance. But don't get me wrong, this mathematical marital advice is not about manipulating the other person. It is about being aware of a pattern in your relationship, bringing it out into the open, and finding a way to resolution. And the beauty with polarisation issues is that resolving them doesn't have to involve fancy fandangled processes. Something as simple and possibly as silly as tossing a coin can do the trick—a great reminder that sometimes our search for sophistication is more a habit than a useful endeavour.

How much sex can you fit in a bean jar?

Isn't it about time we discussed the all-important topic of marital sex? And more importantly how much of it goes on? This is such a minefield. Whole hours of fun rest on the pitiful state of sexual relations within marriage. I mean, what would Woody Allen's career be without it? The following may not be 'Woody Allen', but you might still have come across it:

> Starting on your wedding night and continuing through the first year of your marriage, put one bean in a jar every time you have sex. Starting with the beginning of your second year of marriage, take one bean out of the jar every time you have sex. When you die there will be some beans left in the jar!

I don't know if you can relate to this, but could it really be true? I mean, if your sex life did go along such lines, how much sex could you expect after two, ten or fifty years? Maybe it remains steady throughout the years at one-hundredth the amount you had in the first. Maybe in the second year you can look forward to half the amount of sex you had in the first but then close to none afterwards. What *is* this theory really saying? We *need* to know. In 1970, the mathematician J. David Martin kindly addressed this very issue. Don't tell me mathematicians don't have a sense of humour!

First, he rewrote the 'bean jar sex theory' mathematically as:

$$C_1 > C_2 + C_3 + \cdots + C_n \, ,$$

where C stands for 'coital event'. If you wish to work on this formula, feel free to choose a symbol of your own devising. And don't think this is out of your realm. There isn't any wild mathematics here. This formula just says the number of times you'll have sex in your first year of marriage will be more than the sum of all the times you have sex after that.

Each year your number of sexual encounters has the potential to change. The suggestion is it declines at some rate, be it big or small, as the years go by. The next step is to describe a way in which it does this so as to end up with some beans left in the jar after twenty, thirty, or fifty years of marriage, say. This could happen in a variety of ways. For example, your number of sexual encounters could decline gradually and uniformly throughout your married life. Or, it could decline rapidly in the first two years and then taper to an extremely slow decline by the time you are in your fortieth year of partnership. All the different ways this can happen dictate how the number of romantic interludes peters out as the years go by. Martin examined some of the standard options.

To make the numbers tractable, and to leave some hope for sexual encounters in later years, he started with an admittedly high rate of 1000 coital events in the first year. You'd have to be pretty industrious to reach that level I'd say. But then I could be admitting to an inadequacy. In any case, Martin calculated bean jar sex theory bonking rates for the years following marriage, based on various rates of decline. Here's an example. After that first amazing year, you could sustain 49 sexual encounters a year in a twenty-year marriage and end up with beans left in the jar. But does that sound realistic? Going from 1000 to 49 bonks in one year is equivalent to a 95.1 per cent drop in sexual activity. Now I know the prevailing assumption is marital sex becomes sad, but that's going a bit far.

What if each year your number of bonks was half the number you had the year before. Then in your eleventh year of marriage you would bonk once, and then you would say goodbye to the activity altogether. That doesn't sound right either, does it? But having sex each year by an amount that is half the amount of the previous year represents quite an intense drop-off rate. For Martin, the most plausible bean jar sex theory model he found incorporated an overall softer drop in the number of sexual encounters. But even then, to end up with beans left in the jar means in your second year of marriage you would again be having less than 5 per cent of the amount of sex you were enjoying in the first. In other words, you would go from having 1000 bonks to having less than 50 in one year. You'd be hoping there was a good movie to watch on TV the night of your first wedding anniversary, wouldn't you? It doesn't really make sense. And like this, Martin kept coming up against this brick wall: no matter which decline he looked at, the end result was completely unrealistic. The bean jar sex theory just couldn't be made to work in a marriage of any reasonable length.

Martin tried an adaptation. What if you filled your sex jar for two years before starting to take the beans out? Does that describe any sort of married sex life? Better, but nope, and in fact it turns to worse if you don't reach those 1000 bonks in your first year. Now the results do reflect to an extent what Martin deems to be a plausible marital sex life. And coming from a mathematician, you may see this as a real worry. But I think it is still safe to say, when it comes to sex, best to leave your beans and jars out of it.

Glad I don't have to worry about that predicament anymore. But there is an intellectually serious ending to this story because being able to predict how much sex goes on in marriage has many important uses: from calculating how long a woman is unable to conceive after childbirth (which naturally depends on how much sex she is having), to understanding the evolution of certain diseases (like cervical cancer), to finding out if there is a link between the amount of sex being had and harmony within relationships. And the simple solution of asking thousands of couples to keep sex diaries doesn't appear to work. Yes, one reason is because people have a tendency to lie about this topic. But as Mary Rogers Gillmore from the University of Washington with some of her colleagues showed in 2001, getting people to record their every sexual move seems particularly susceptible to a number of other more subtle problems. One is the self-monitoring effect, which is where people start to change their behaviour as they develop an awareness of it. Another is the fatigue effect, which is where no matter what behaviour is being recorded its frequency tends to decay over time. And whether these two effects are completely dissociated is another aspect of the discussion.

Also, some of the studies I read where couples had contributed sex diaries, began with a disclaimer noting the results of the work could in fact only apply to people with obsessive-compulsive personalities—the types required to keep such records! Finding out how much bonking is going on out there is very hard work.

And if you can't rely on sex diaries, what can you do? Well, predict bonking rates with mathematics. The bean jar sex theory may not work, but there is bound to be another theory that does. There is a marital sex equation out there. We just have to find it. Any volunteers?

$$\partial x / \partial x + \partial x / \partial x + \partial x / \partial x + \partial x / \partial x + \partial x / \partial x + \partial x / \partial x + \partial x / \partial x$$

Marriage is a really tricky one. It is something emotional, psychological and cultural all at once. Even economics and politics come into it, with tax and divorce laws having a significant effect on marriage trends in society. And the term 'marriage' seems a little restrictive these days, doesn't it. What about the de-facto relationships, gay and lesbian relationships, and open marriages: we've only just begun studying our 'pair bonding' from these many different perspectives. And the intricate manner in which people interact, connect and influence each other makes it feel so right to have mathematics involved. It couldn't be more about patterns if we tried!

We've just been given three mathematical tips to play with. Tell me, are you going to start watching out for how much you compromise? Begin keeping an eye out for issues of polarisation? And stop listening to people when they tell you how much sex you're supposed to be having? But wait, there's more! Patterns exist in many forms and ones leading to mathematical marital tips are but one aspect of the problem. To highlight the complexity of our pair bonding, let me finish with an interesting complication raised by two economists, Bruno Frey and Reiner Eichenberger, in 1996. It has to do with our patterns of logic.

A basic premise in economics is that people act as best they can to reach their preferred agenda. And in many economic models these days, where family is seen as an integral part of the economy, agendas include items such as marrying, having children, or setting money aside for loved ones. Remember utility functions in polarisation? Utility functions characterised the worth of something to someone. To build models of the economy, economists use utility functions to consider the worth of people's agendas. They then consider rules of logic dictating how people will pursue these agendas. The mathematics of utility functions is the mathematics of 'common sense and particular agendas'.

And here is where Bruno Frey and Reiner Eichenberger noticed an interesting twist. When it comes to marriage it seems our logical reasoning goes funny. I began the chapter by noting how many of us choose to ignore the high odds of divorce. Which is quite amazing when you think about what we are putting on the line: isn't it our life? It's not just risking a couple of dollars in a lottery. And we don't stop there with our bizarre logic. When we make a big purchase, like a car, don't we seek advice? We get input from magazines and books and friends and family? Yes. But when it comes to relationships, we hardly do, if at all. In fact asking for advice somehow feels wrong. If it is love, there's no guesswork or advice needed—it just has to 'feel right'. Marriage is supposed to be based on romance and love, and these subjective qualities aren't to be reasoned with. Rule number one: avoid rational advice. Which brings in another logic issue, why do we insist on basing our marital choices on passionate love when research shows we know full well passion is the first victim of familiarity? What are we doing? Actively courting disaster? Traditionally, people learn from their mistakes, but not in this area it seems. After a first divorce, most people remarry, even in the face of a higher divorce rate . . . and they do so relatively quickly. I do exclude arranged marriages here, but that's because the individuals themselves aren't playing the strategy game so it's a completely different area altogether.

Now psychologists, sociologists and other marriage experts are busily finding ways for us to rectify our wacky logic, but for economist like Bruno Frey and Reiner Eichenberger the key is not to try and change it but to embrace it so economic models become more accurate. And, call me crazy, but they may have a point. Maybe if we clarified our utility functions when it comes to marriage, we would find our rules of logic fit quite perfectly. What is it that we are really after in marriage? If it's to indulge in fanciful, passionate emotions then isn't it wackiness that we're after in the first place? Our paradoxical behaviour could be quite justified. Oh, dear, I'm getting way too philosophical again. But this is what all this mathematics brings out in me. Giving a mathematical context to our behaviours when approaching marriage or when in marriage is like handing me a marital weather map. I see a large formation of patterns of all colours; I see highs, lows, storms and balmy weather evolving everywhere; it becomes less about the patterns themselves and more about the beauty of navigating through the complex, evolving mix. Instead of just searching for answers, or questioning what's right versus what's wrong, mathematics is a great way to consider how everything works as a whole.

Chapter 3

ROAD TESTING THE BED
HOW MUCH SEX IS TOO MUCH SEX?

I never know when to drop a lover, do you? Is it fair to expect intellectual, physical and emotional satiation by the one person? If not, how much should you compromise? If you are physically and emotionally stimulated, as a mark of two out of three, is that great or not enough? If you meet someone and things are going really, really, great, how do you know you won't meet someone where things will go really, really, really, great? I know some say: 'you just know'. Hmmm. OK, maybe you will. In the meantime a little mathematics can tell you when you're suffering from a severe case of 'the grass is always greener'.

Every now and then, I look back at my series of short to long-term relationships and do a relationship audit. Maybe I should have persevered with so-and-so . . . flashback—ooo, no.

Maybe I just don't like being in a relationship full stop. How many lovers should I have before I can feel reasonably confident I've at least had *the possibility* of 'happily ever after'?

It's time for an exotic Middle Eastern tale . . .

In a kingdom far, far, away a sultan has been questioning the true wisdom of his chief adviser and so decides to set him a test. Knowing the adviser is seeking a wife, the sultan arranges for one hundred intelligent and beautiful women to be brought before him in succession. The adviser's task is to pick the woman with the highest dowry. If he picks correctly, he gets to marry that woman, and keep his post. If not, he gets his head chopped off. The adviser obviously finds himself in a grave situation.

The women are to present themselves to the adviser one at a time and reveal their dowry to him. At each introduction he must decide immediately if that woman has the highest dowry out of the one hundred, or he must let her pass. The adviser has no idea of the range of dowries before he starts and cannot return to any woman he rejects. Once he lets them go, they are gone forever. The adviser begins to wonder if the wife thing is worth it, but it's too late. The sultan has cornered him and he has to make a choice. Is there anything he can possibly do to increase his chance of picking the woman with the highest dowry and keep his head?

His true wisdom will be revealed if he turns to mathematics to help him out, because mathematics has the answer. A couple of pages of sums looking like this one

$$\pi(s,n) = \frac{1}{n} \sum_{k=s}^{n} \frac{s-1}{k-1},$$

give the perfect strategy.

This is what the sums suggest the adviser should do: he should check and reject the first thirty-seven women, no matter what, but make a note of the highest dowry he comes across in this group; then starting with the thirty-eighth woman he should pick the first woman he meets whose dowry is higher than the highest dowry from the first group. Done deal. This is how he will maximise his chance of picking correctly. Now sure, there is a possibility he might have already rejected the woman with the highest dowry as part of the initial thirty-seven women. Or that he might pick a woman too soon. But this is his best option, loaded with a 37 per cent chance of success. Which might not sound too flash, but that amounts to being correct over a third of the time, so it's not too un-flash either. And it is a darn sight better than the 1 per cent chance he has of winning if he just guessed.

OK. So much for the adviser finding his perfect mate. How about us? Is there a mathematical strategy we can use to increase our chance of finding the love of our life? Peter Todd from the Max Planck Institute for Psychological Research in Germany has shown how this fable is a source of advice for our lonely souls as well. Now, I know, I know, we are not all chief advisers being presented with potential partners on a platter. And I personally long for the day when my choice of lover rests on something as concrete and straight forward as a dowry. But as Todd points out, there are really only two things separating us ordinary people from the chief adviser's position. Well, three, if you count having your head chopped off for picking the wrong one. Which, come to think of it, might sound more appealing than living the misery of being in the wrong relationship. Anyway . . . I digress . . .

What are the main differences between our partner search and the chief adviser's? First, we don't know how many potential partners we are likely to meet. Second, we don't really need to pick '*the* best' to live happily ever after. More than likely we probably don't even know what 'the best' is. We have some idea of our likes and dislikes and we can more or less order these by importance. But let's face it, most of us would be happy to settle down with someone sitting in the top 10 or even 25 per cent—especially if in the long run this means experiencing significantly less lonely nights.

With these minor adjustments, how does the strategy change? How many potential partners—or let's be candid and say, how many lovers—should we cruise through before settling down with reasonable confidence we have made a good choice? Or alternatively, be able to settle back with a chuffed look on our face, cognac in hand, and say: 'You know, I could have if I'd wanted to.'

Well, the answer is that a dozen should do the trick! Sleep with twelve people. Then settle down with the next best that comes along. Seems achievable. And this gives you over 75 per cent chance of success, depending on your standards. Of course, sleeping with more people in that initial sample is always good, but it is worth knowing the mathematics says more than about thirty and you're over-researching. Which can also be good, sure. Just don't kid yourself!

Maybe you have wanted to settle down for a while now and you are feeling desperate. Would you be happy to settle with someone who simply wasn't in the *bottom* 25 per cent? Then Todd has a strategy for you too. Personally, if you have reached such a stage, I would suggest you try going to your local bar in a bikini and see what happens—but that tactic might have a female bias. What does Todd have to say? Sleep with between two and ten people and settle with the best after that. 'The best' here meaning someone who is not in your bottom 25 per cent bracket.

Yes, all these figures are very rough and of course our individual lives and experiences come into play. For one, I have described the problem with a bit of a personal bias: you don't really have to *sleep* with twelve people and then start the search, *dating* is fine; likewise, one-night stands probably shouldn't count. It is all about deciding who has the best qualities for you. Todd's calculations assume we will meet anywhere between a hundred and a thousand potentials over the course of our lifetime. Just think of all the people you meet at work, at the store or actually out on the prowl at your favourite club. Now decide on your criteria. Do you think you could potentially sleep with a hundred or more people in your life? Do you think you could potentially meet a hundred or more people who would set your heart on fire with their conversation? Whatever you decide upon, it is reassuring to know you can quite conceivably find a beautiful partner without having to road test the hundreds beforehand. All you have to do is test twelve and pick the best after that. I'll refer to it as the 'have a dozen test-bonks' strategy or the 'twelve-bonk rule' for short.

Now all this might seem particularly tailored for singles on the lookout, however there are some wider implications to Todd's study, and they specifically concern people who have already picked a life partner. Remember our high divorce rates? Well, they have people theorising all over the place. What are we doing when partner-picking? Are we creatures made for serial monogamy? Could we be trying to attempt the impossible with life-lasting relationships? Or maybe we just don't work hard enough when we have the possibility of one? Do we pair up for all the wrong reasons? Or do we simply not search for a partner long enough? This last question is not without merit. Turns out, about a third of people still marry their childhood sweetheart. Which prompts the question of whether we use a search strategy at all. And if we do search, the question still remains, how long should a search run for in order to be considered 'long enough'?

These questions were in fact Todd's motivation for his study. He wanted to unearth the search strategies people could actually be using and how long they would take for successful implementation. Now, people would not necessarily be using these strategies consciously. The strategies would more than likely be lurking in our genetic make-up, having evolved over tens of thousands of years.

Todd's adaptation of the 'sultan and chief adviser' problem turned out to be a very plausible strategy. As we saw, this was a mathematically tested optimal approach, and meant cruising through a dozen people before looking for your perfect match. Seemingly a far cry from hooking up with your childhood sweetheart, but there is more to the story. Recall how Todd's calculations assume we will meet anywhere between a hundred and a thousand potentials over the course of our lifetime. As Todd points out, being able to choose from such large numbers is a relatively new experience for us. Not so long ago, we were confined to our local area, village or tribe, whose size remained constant and fairly small. When you reduce your sample to such small sizes, turns out hooking up with your childhood sweetheart is not such a bad strategy after all. Maybe we are failing at mate searching today because we are using an outdated 50 000-year-old strategy: the 'have *a* test-bonk' strategy. We might have been well adapted to our environment once, but it has changed considerably and quickly. And we're just not up to speed. We need to upgrade to the dozen.

Another reason why Todd's 'have a dozen test-bonks' strategy could very well be the one we use subconsiously is that it's simple, easily applicable and gives good results. And this complements latest theories on how our brains work with heuristics. You know, rules of thumb, like the one where if the video cover shows a beautiful bikini-clad woman pointing a gun, then the movie's a dud.

Back in the '50s, it was thought our brains echoed perfect mathematical techniques. A beautiful mathematical solution to a problem might take pages of work, but our brains were thought to churn through it in a flash. With the invention of computers and their ability to do exactly that, churn through amazing mathematical calculations at lightning speed, we have been surprised to find out we still can't get computers to perform like we do. We appear to have a capacity to discard information, to adapt, to sift out irrelevancies, and to cope with much larger amounts of data. We seem to obey 'rules of thumb'. And in practice our rule of thumb results are often close to the mathematical optimum anyway. Todd's 'have a dozen test-bonks' strategy is an illustration of these ideas.

So while, over the years, researchers have examined a number of other mathematical search strategies for how we might mate search, because these are so much more complicated than Todd's, they are not as likely to be representative of how our minds actually tick. Some take into account the cost of searching—not just 'dinner and movie' bills but emotional costs also. Others take into account the fact that as we search we learn about what is available and might change the priorities on our 'likes and dislikes' list. But all these strategies just take too long and require too much knowledge about the partners. And they also require considerably greater mathematics. Which I realise might be a scary thought for some, but there's no need to worry—the extra mathematics would be performed subconsciously by the brain.

Todd's mathematics offers a lot: a method for single people to find a life partner, as well as reasons for why so many paired people end up single again.

And now a few other search options . . .

Enough of what can fit comfortably into the nature of things. Now we know the basic model, if we really want to get into it, there are optional added features. Here are a couple.

How is your conscience about having an affair?

Affairs give you the possibility of holding on to one person while still testing for better options, or in other words, 'keeping your options open'. I've also heard this referred to as practising the 'monkey grip'—you swing from branch to branch, not letting go until you have the other tightly gripped.

To study affairs we are forced back to the ideal case of the sultan's adviser, because that's where most of the mathematics has been performed. However, when we slacken the sultan's rules a little 'à la Todd' to fit them to our situation, it looks like we're in for a better average for much less searching anyway.

The adviser had a 37 per cent chance of picking the woman with the highest dowry. John Gilbert and Frederick Mosteller showed back in 1966 that if he could keep hold of one woman while still continuing his search, his chances of picking the right woman would increase to 60 per cent. In our case, this amounts to having an affair. OK, if the mathematics says so?!?! What else does the mathematics say? The more women the chief adviser can keep hold of, the better his odds get. If he could keep seven women and still search for an eighth, his chances of picking the right woman would sky rocket to 96 per cent.

Does this mean if we can juggle eight lovers at once our chances of finding true love increase substantially? Forget about your conscience, the simple fact that there are only seven days in a week should be enough of a deterrent. I don't know about you, but in more frivolous times in my life I have dabbled in such activities (never made it up to eight though, sorry to disappoint). What a mess! It is said breaking up, losing a loved one, and spending time in jail are the top most stressful experiences. Excuse me I don't think so: try remembering at least two versions of every story of what you did the night before, having no spare time and incorporating extra showers into your already busy day.

I think here we are staring at a great project where the maths should be expanded to include emotional and psychological costs—some future research to look forward to. In the mean time though, if you're game, go for it!

Are you the sex object everyone is drawn to?

Then, you might have thought Todd's assumption you couldn't return to potentials gone by a little presumptuous. Don't worry. People like Canadian university professor Ruth Corbin have looked into this in some detail. She has studied a number of scenarios concerning your chances of being able to waltz back into someone's life. Now, if you are Brad Pitt, then you might always be able to do that, but for most of us our qualities only carry us so far. Have you stayed on good terms with your exes? Maybe you sustain a 50 per cent chance of being able to return to an ex, maybe your chances decrease steadily as years go by, maybe they stay high for some time but then drop off suddenly (as they each get married, for example). Corbin put all these perspectives through a mathematical blender and found a whole host of theorems like this one:

> Theorem: Suppose $N > k > 0$. After k observations have been made, if $\alpha(0)/k > \alpha(t_k) - \alpha(t_k + 1)$ then $V^c[k, t_k] > V^s[k, t_k]$. That is, the better strategy is to continue to make observations.

What I like is the end result, which basically amounts to: push your luck as far as you can! It is reassuring to find mathematics hasn't missed the point.

While Todd's analysis came up with the 'have a dozen test-partners before settling down' strategy, Corbin's analysis says if you think the option to pick a past one is there, then hold off and search for longer before settling down. You can always try to exercise that option later. Yes, this might not work, but it's all about how to increase your likelihood of picking the best lover your life has to offer. And the higher your chances of picking a past potential as your final choice, the more your search should be extended. Think of the extreme case where you could return to any you felt like: you could extend your search to test all partners you think possible and then simply sit back in front of your smorgasbord and make a choice.

The sad reality is, though, our chances of returning to an ex will more than likely change over the years. And mathematically the way to deal with this is to stop searching and prepare to pick your soul mate as soon as you see your chances start to diminish. Yet there is one interesting, maybe unexpected, result mathematics uncovers. If you find your chance of picking a past lover only decreases by a fixed amount each time you get a new one, then theorems say you should push your luck and behave as if you were a sex god and could return to any lover at any time. This is where you test all partners you think possible and then choose from the smorgasbord. Of course working out this 'fixed amount' is another matter. Some severe mathematical modelling will be required to even find out if it is lurking in your love life. But hey, if you think you can see the pattern, why not throw caution to the wind, strut your stuff and keep testing partners till you've had enough! (Got to be a song title in there somewhere.)

Want the deluxe model?

Be prepared for some serious work. If you think dressing sexy and brushing up on the latest news or gossip so you appear hot and brainy is too much effort, wait till you see what this involves.

The idea is neat. The basic search strategy is modified a little so we maximise the quality of what we pick, rather than maximise our chances of picking quality. An interesting twist studied since the '60s.

As usual, you should begin by sampling a number of potential partners and then start looking for 'the one'. If that special someone hasn't appeared after a fixed number of lovers, then you should drop your standards a little and start looking for 'the one' and anything close. Then if that special someone still hasn't appeared after another fixed number of lovers, you should drop your standards a little further and start looking for 'the one', anything close and anything close to anything close. You catch my drift. Continue the process of every now and then dropping your standards and eventually you'll end up with something! (Maybe that was the technique 89-year-old oil tycoon J. Howard Marshall used when he married Anna Nicole Smith. Still single at his age, had his standards dropped to the point where they included only one item: 'large breasts'?!)

The hard work is finding out when it's time to drop your standards. The mathematics is quite complex. So much so, the calculations have only been performed for a limited number of cases. In 1996, Malcolm Quine and J. Law working at the University of Sydney in Australia found 'standard dropping' times for when you could be sure to meet up to a hundred potential lovers in a lifetime and were only prepared to let your standards drop three times. Never mind extending the mathematics to deal with your particular situation, just finding the information needed to use the mathematics seems like a lot of hard work. You have to find exactly how many potential lovers you think you will come across in your life and combine that with how many you are prepared to have a go with. Then you have to decide how many times you will drop your standards. I'm already thinking I'd rather go to the pub in a bikini and see what happens.

In 1980, Arthur Frank and Stephen Samuels from Purdue University in the US considered the situation where, during the course of your life, you have an infinite number of potential lovers at your disposal. Not just a case study good for the ego, but also good for the mathematics as it simplifies. Well, it becomes as simple as:

$$Q_r > 2^{-r} \text{ for all } r = 1,2\ldots \text{ and for all } t \in (0,1)$$

$$\limsup Q_r(t)^{1/r} \leq \inf_{0 \leq \alpha \leq t} \max\left\{ t^{\alpha}, \left(\frac{t}{\alpha}\right)^{\alpha}\left(\frac{1-t}{1-\alpha}\right)^{1-\alpha} \right\}$$

Not something you'll find on any high school mathematics curriculum. However theorems like these expose some of the broad features of the advanced search and partially light the pathway to more specific results.

Here is how the advanced search fares out. As usual, begin by simply testing a fixed number of potential soul mates. I'd pick the twelve Todd suggested with his research. Then if you are happy to let your standards go really low eventually, look a little bit further, like a couple of people, and if you don't find what you are after, drop your standards a little. Test a couple more people and if 'soul mate' still hasn't come your way, drop your standards a little further. And so on.

If you are somewhat fussy and don't want to let your standards drop too much, do the same thing but have a go with more people between each 'standard drop', like maybe half a dozen or less if you started with the twelve. The more you are willing to drop your standards, the less number of people you should play with each time.

And keep in mind the following extras. The first group of potential soul mates you have a go with should be your biggest test sample. The ground you gain by dropping your standards each time is large, so don't plan on going too far. And always practise safe sex . . . I should have said that earlier, shouldn't I?

I don't know how well this advanced search method could be incorporated into a daily routine. Most researchers also reject the notion of it being part of our genetic set-up. It does seem unlikely our brains would have evolved to be so sophisticated as to work subconsciously through theorems like the one above. Much more likely for them to have developed a strategy like the one Todd suggested: test a fixed amount and that's it. But, I don't know, I don't want to reject this hypothesis so readily. Maybe we have caught ourselves out in the midst of development, on our way to becoming perfect subconscious mathematical analysts. If we let evolution take its course, we might find our brains do eventually evaluate such complex theorems to help us find partners. I say this not just because I have a perverse desire everyone will one day find out they are in fact mathematicians, but because something rings very familiar. For those of us who haven't married our childhood sweethearts, there definitely is a sensation of a more realistic approach to love. Childhood dreams of that perfect someone vanish throughout puberty and our early twenties. People who are still single in their thirties always speak of compromise and effort as key components of relationships. Isn't that a softer, more fancy way of saying 'a dropping of standards'?

$$\partial x / \partial x + \partial x / \partial x + \partial x / \partial x + \partial x / \partial x + \partial x / \partial x + \partial x / \partial x + \partial x / \partial x$$

I haven't actually counted, but I am more than pretty sure I've had more than twelve lovers. Woohoo! Though I'm definitely sure I haven't made the magic twelve when it comes to falling in love, not even close. So the real work is deciding how to approach Todd's study. Is it the 'twelve-bonk rule' for you? And if so, who are you going to count as part of those initial twelve? The ones you are still friends with? The ones you swore you would have died for? Or simply the ones your mother liked?

Now if your criteria does involve lover counting make sure you're meticulous because when it comes to number of lovers, a little mathematical incongruity shows we have a tendency to be a bit all over the shop. Men report having bonked on average two to four times as many women as women do men. Since they're bonking each other here, someone's telling fibs. But do they know they are? The latest research by Norman Brown and Robert Sinclair from the University of Alberta in Canada suggests it might actually be the strategy used to come up with those numbers that is at fault. They have evidence women prefer to enumerate all their past lovers while men have a tendency to resort to making rough approximations. A woman is likely to count through the names: 'Brad, Tom, Justin, the one with the nice arms . . . ' but a man is likely to say 'about twenty a year, for three years . . . '. And enumeration is prone to an underestimation of achievements, while approximation is prone to an overestimation. Women probably feel a bit of societal pressure to take their sexual activities more seriously than men and so may be more prepared to put in the extra effort required for the enumeration technique. Nevertheless both techniques are imperfect and global average lover numbers can't be announced with any real accuracy as yet.

But we are brought back to the importance of strategy, which is really what the 'twelve-bonk rule' is getting at. Choosing the right strategy to solve a problem can have a huge effect on the solution. It is all about focusing on the journey, not the destination. Peter Todd's motivation for the 'twelve-bonk rule' was to find an example of a simple strategy that gives good results. And mate searching is but the tip of the iceberg. He works closely with Gerd Gigerenzer as part of a group of researchers really focusing their efforts on finding more of these types of strategies. Not only may they hold the key to how our minds work, but 'simplicity' translates into 'rapidity', and is crucial in many environments like hospital emergency rooms or the stock market.

We can look at these strategies some other time but for the time being I think we can milk the 'twelve-bonk rule' or the 'take the next-best idea' for a while. Looking for a parking spot? Think of an area in the vicinity of your destination and then 'bang', pick the first spot that comes after that. No questions asked. Looking for the best flatmate? Interview and reject twelve and then 'wham', pick the next best that comes along. Looking through assorted chocolates for the one you are going to have? Try twelve then pick the next best after that. Hey, have I got the theory right?!

Chapter 4

DATING SERVICES
ARE YOU REALLY BEING SERVED?

My experience is, no matter how cynical or world-weary we become, there is always a part of us drawn to the destiny-ridden notion of being on a collision course with a pre-prepared soul mate. Somewhere out there in the universe, a one-only, the one that was meant to be. But, whenever someone engages with a dating service, this fateful notion is put aside, at least temporarily. With dating services we want our romantic ideal to be orchestrated by somebody else, hopefully using fail-safe scientific principles. And, yes, many of us do want this service. Dating services have been listed as one of the 100 best new businesses of the 1990s (Bulcroft et al. 2000). If you have ever looked up 'dating service' in the phone book or on the web, you will know there are absolutely millions of such businesses out there. And you will also know they have a tendency to use words like 'computerised matching' or 'advanced computer technology'. That's where the scientific principles come in. What that jargon is short for is 'someone has analysed a problem, found the essential components, worked out how they fit together and therefore how to solve it, and has then set up a mechanical device to perform the task on any scale, tirelessly, over and over again'. Now if this is done properly it will require loads of mathematics. And, in a field as complex as finding decent relationships, the more mathematics the better! So, what do dating services get up to?

Dating services are pools of data. You fill in reams of questionnaires aimed at revealing your entire soul. Questions such as: What religion are you? What colour eyes do you have? What is your political persuasion? What movies do you like? Do you like your partners to have table manners? Dating services enter this data into a computer that performs the mechanical tasks I referred to above. Out comes a list of people as similar to you and your envisioned ideal partner as possible. The computer searches: similar interests, personality, beliefs etc. The service then introduces you. Similarity appears to be a good bet for a true love match, which I'll delve into further in Chapter 6.

As preliminary research for this chapter, it was compulsory for me to join a few dating services. That's my excuse anyway, and I'm sticking with it. Though I've always been extremely curious about just who I would meet through such means. And with the Internet, it is just so easy and non-threatening. You log on, fill in a questionnaire, get given a special email address, and after receiving some suggested matches, or sometimes after browsing through a myriad profiles, you email the potentials.

Potential what? That's up to you. The point is we've become so accustomed to email relationships in general I think making contact with someone through an agency doesn't feel as full-on as it might have before. Today, there are bars, gyms, and cyberspace. And with cyberspace, we don't have to fear coming into contact with the stereotyped dating service consultant: the rotund woman with highly teased hair and acrylic nails. All in all, if you haven't had a taste, watch out, Internet dating services are fun and addictive! Well, unless you get the ultimate fix—a romantic collision.

So how do these services build a client profile? What types of questions do they ask? How many questions does it take for them to have you classified? Here are some examples.

The famous US-based service found at www.matchmaker.com needs some fifty questions and twenty-three small essays about yourself to do the trick. Sounds like you could end up in a self-analysis coma, but I found myself laughing out loud. The service has a fun feel to it. Here are a couple of their questions:

How would you describe your physique?

- ○ Chiselled, I work out every day!
- ○ Toned, I keep fit
- ○ 'Height–weight' proportionate
- ○ Skinny, I could use some carbohydrates
- ○ Voluptuous/Portly
- ○ Large but shapely
- ○ Rotund
- ○ I look like a reflection in a fun-house mirror!

Which is your favorite season?

○ Winter
○ Spring
○ Summer
○ Fall
○ Football

Matchmaker.com is huge. They boast of having well over five million registered members with more than 50 000 members joining weekly.

Another US-based service having received some attention is Matchupsingles.com (www.matchupsingles.com). While Matchupsingles.com obviously doesn't aim for the same fun feel as Matchmaker.com, some of their ninety-six questions leave you wondering:

When it comes to parties:

○ I am not a herd animal
○ Holiday celebrations only
○ I enjoy an occasional small one with good friends
○ Large or small, I like them all

Being 'In Love' is:

○ Just an excuse for sex
○ Of no importance in selecting a mate
○ Something that fades in time. The love you earn is the love that lasts
○ Critical to happiness in marriage

Matchupsingles.com even gives you a choice on the income level of your preferred match. One option is to be matched with only people whose income is 'less than US$25 000'. Doesn't that sound like bordering on a fetish?

Then there is the popular Australian-based service found at www.rsvp.com.au. RSVP reports having about 200 000 members. This smaller membership might be why a basic partner search can be achieved with some fifteen questions. Can this really be enough information to perform people matching? Well, we'll soon see limited information doesn't necessarily mean the match will be less efficient.

So how does it work? How do dating services actually calculate how similar we are to someone? Well, the exact answer to that question is I haven't the foggiest. They're such big businesses, and there is so much money involved, they don't publish their secrets. And each company will have its own specific methods anyway. But I'm not completely in the dark. After all, Coca-Cola and Pepsi don't publish their recipes, yet you don't have to be a chemist or need a lab to work out both these drinks contain a hell of a lot of sugar and caffeine. And similarly, I know one mathematical ingredient dating services must deal with in their calculations: *the curse of dimensionality*. I'm not making that name up. It might sound like the latest horror movie by Wes Craven, but that's just what it's called round the traps. A famous Brooklyn-born contributor of mathematical ideas, Richard Bellman coined the term in a book he published in 1961. And it certainly lives up to its name: it has given considerable grief and shows no sign of relenting. Today, a major area of research is devoted to working out how to break the dreaded dimensionality curse, and what the repercussions are. Forget about teased hair and acrylic nails, the modern dating service consultant is bound to have bottle-top glasses and an obsessive love of Star Trek—aren't these the classic afflictions of those who have stared at a computer screen for days on end?

Similarity and the curse of dimensionality

Finding your ideal partner using a bunch of questions requires a field of mathematics called higher dimensional arithmetic. The important thing to keep in mind is a dimension is just an aspect or trait. That's one of the standard definitions you'll find in the dictionary. A dimension doesn't have to be of the spatial type, as in the typical Star Trek plot where the Starship Enterprise warps off into another dimension. It is more like in advertising when they say, 'Sexy Shampoo will add dimension to your hair'. Your hair can't suddenly be seen in another dimension! What they really mean is Sexy Shampoo will bring a new feature to your hair, or add something extra, another aspect or trait. So if you answer fifty questions for a dating service, you have described yourself with fifty traits. A mathematician would immediately see that as a fifty dimensional scenario. The picture will become clearer as we go further. And, don't forget the curse awaits us!

Let's start with an apparently simple but typical case. Say a dating service asked the four questions below, each with three possible answers:

	1 Hate	2 No strong opinion	3 Thoroughly adore
Q1) What do you think of smoking?	❏	❏	❏
Q2) Do you like visiting museums?	❏	❏	❏
Q3) How do you feel about astrology?	❏	❏	❏
Q4) Do you like to have sex with work colleagues?	❏	❏	❏

Along come James, Fran and Sue with their answers:

	James	Fran	Sue
Q1)	1	1	3
Q2)	1	3	1
Q3)	1	2	1
Q4)	1	2	3

If you're in the mood, add yourself into the mix. The question we're asking is: Who is James more similar to, Fran or Sue? Or you, if you like. One way to answer this question is to simply add up all the differences between two people's answers:

James and Fran differ by 2 on Q2, 1 on Q3, and 1 on Q4. That gives a difference of 4.

James and Sue differ by 2 on Q1 and 2 on Q4. That also gives a difference of 4.

Here is an interesting point. James is measured to be as similar to Fran as he is to Sue, but Fran and Sue have quite different tastes. Sue sees eye to eye with James on two items: museums and astrology. But then she is his opposite when it comes to smoking and having sex with work colleagues. On the other hand, Fran differs strongly to James only on one item: museum visiting. Her other differences are only mild. Surely there must be a way to discriminate between these two lasses for James?

There is another way to measure similarity. You square the differences before you add them up. This means if there's a difference of 2, that counts as $2^2 = 4$. The effect of the squaring process is to make larger differences count more than smaller ones. Larger numbers get much bigger than smaller numbers when they're squared. So what does this mean for James?

James and Fran count their differences as $2^2 + 1^2 + 1^2 = 6$

James and Sue count their differences as $2^2 + 2^2 = 8$

This looks promising: 6 is smaller than 8. Fran has more in common with James than Sue does. Problem solved. Fran and James should go out on a date.

The aim of this little bit of mostly painless mathematics was to show you how similarity is all a matter of the way you decide to count the differences. And you can choose to do that in any which way your heart desires. It can be as basic or as complicated as you wish. A favourite among mathematicians is to use the formula:

$$d_\tau(p, q) = \left(\sum_{i=1}^{D} |p_i - q_i|^\tau \right)^{1/\tau} .$$

Do you think this looks messy? What's the favourite formula among dating services then? I doubt if it looks that simple! One of their jobs is to decide which one they are going to use from the many possibilities. In effect, they choose who should be with who. Change the method and it is quite likely your perfect match will change too. Life in the dating service world is not as simple as it first appears.

I will give you some idea of how dating services might pick their formula a little further down the track. But we've reached a stage where a couple of things should be mentioned. First, I must highlight the level of sophistication of the mathematics we have just done. The calculations might be straightforward but the ideas are pretty hardcore. We were working with 4 questions—that is, 4 dimensions—and believe it or not, we were calculating the difference between two objects in 4 dimensions. Yes, I've just had you calculating distances in 4 dimensions. Move aside Einstein, we're on a roll!

But, here is my second thing: this all works until we're confronted with *the curse of dimensionality*. It turns out the more questions there are, or in other words the more dimensions you take into consideration, the harder it can be to find a concept of similarity that makes sense. Why? Because all calculated differences can end up being around the same number. The difference between the differences can be so small that how different you are to someone or similar to them becomes open to many interpretations. Cause for confusion? Let me explain.

With our last calculations, James and Fran counted their differences as 6 and James and Sue as 8. Fran is 2 'steps' closer to James than Sue is. Now imagine a database, like some of these agencies have, with thousands, even millions of people. And imagine calculating who's the person with the least differences to you, and who the most. In other words who is your closest and furthest match. The curse comes into play because the more questions you ask, the more likely the differences between the responses are going to be extremely similar. So similar it could be a bit silly to consider them different. You see, if the difference between you and your closest match is 1000, and the difference between you and your furthest match is 1001, then what does similar really mean? Not forgetting the possibly many medium matches you could have with scores in between 1000 and 1001. If you have a medium match with a score of 1000.1, then wouldn't you want to check them out too? But then what about a medium match with score 1000.11? And 1000.2? And 1000.5? When should you stop? The numbers 1000 to 1001 make for a thin slice on which to base decisions of true love. And the more questions you have, the thinner the slice becomes. It really is a curse. You'd think that the more questions you had, the more information you would have to perform people matching so the better the matches. Instead, the more questions you have, the less matching can make sense. We've arrived at a junction between the fields of mathematics and philosophy. It's about what you *believe* is similar. Well, my philosophy is, 'The glass is always half full'. Everyone can be considered your perfect match. There's a lot of fun to be had, not True Love but Endless Dating. Could this be saying something about our ideal of a predestined soul mate? If joining a dating service can be thought of as bathing in a sea of decent potentials, then could the same be true out in the real world? Maybe I'm getting a little over excited.

We need to know more about this curse. Will it always happen? In 1999, Kevin Beyer, Jonathan Goldstein, Raghu

Ramakrishanan and Uri Shaft, working at the University of Wisconsin-Madison, put forward that it more than likely will. One of the critical factors is the dependency on the set of responses you are trying to compare. If you had a dating service with only mass murderers and heads of religion as clients (bear with me here), then the responses from both groups, being hugely different (hopefully), should lead to people being matched only within their group. Differences should jump out from the results. But in dating services, many people are going to think alike on a number of questions. And the more questions, the harder and harder it becomes to tease out the differences in the data. And for Beyer, Goldstein, Ramakrishanan and Shaft this points to the philosophical disaster of a vanished concept of similarity. Furthermore they found *the curse of dimensionality* could easily take hold with dimensions as few as ten or fifteen. Considering some of the dating services I joined had over ninety questions, this becomes a very pertinent problem.

Some other players prominent in this field of dealing with the curse include Charu Aggarwal from the IBM T. J. Watson Research Center in New York State, and Alexander Hinneburg and Daniel Keim from the University of Halle in Germany. They've worked together to discover if there isn't a way out of the curse's trap. Maybe using a different way to count the differences would have an effect on the curse. This means experimenting with all kinds of formulae like the one above. Could one way of measuring differences show contrast in responses, while others not? If some do, why? And can the contrast be interpreted meaningfully? This is the forefront of current research.

And they do believe there is hope. But I'm not going to start talking about L_∞ *norms, fractional distance metrics* and *noise stability*, because you might prefer to go and read your phone book instead.

You get the point though: finding a closest match requires highly scientific investigations. It is something you have to put a lot of thought into—*a lot*. It is not a simple case of gathering information, whacking it into a computer, and going off to make a cup of tea in the belief that when you return a single answer will be staring out at you from the computer screen.

So what do dating services do?

Dating services do the best they can considering the situation. Faced with the dimensionality problem, dating services have to decide what they believe 'similar' means. They would do this with a series of statistical analyses. And then build their similarity formula. It is not a perfect science. It is more about building as strong a case for similarity as possible. It is about scanning through the data to find some of its key features and seeing if they say anything about what similarity means. And the features dating services would be keeping their eyes open for makes me realise some of the issues I find important in my own relationship shopping:

1) Not every aspect of a person is of equal importance. Say James has a pet snake and enjoys Mexican food. Whether Fran loves Mexican food or not is relatively inconsequential to their match compared to how she feels about snakes. Some things can be compromised on easily, others would require years of

therapy. All the questions dating services ask need to be assessed for such differences in importance. And this then needs to be built into the similarity search:

$$d_\tau(p,q) = \left(\sum_{i=1}^{D} w_i \left| p_i - q_i \right|^\tau \right)^{1/\tau}.$$

2) Many people agree on some questions but fluctuate greatly on others. For example, 'What is your preferred time of the day?' is going to yield all kinds of answers. But 'Do you like to have sex with work colleagues?' is probably going to yield an overwhelming number of 'no's. So 'yes' answers to that question should be flagged. Dating services need to comb through all the answers for such different variations in opinions. And again, build these different variations into the similarity search.

3) Many opinions are interrelated. With a large number of questions answered by thousands or even millions of people, it is likely patterns in the responses will emerge—patterns that may not be self-evident. For example, as you scan through the data you might find people who enjoy walking also enjoy action movies. So for the walkers, movie tastes bring no added value, they can be discarded. But life isn't usually this simple and you are more likely to find more subtle patterns like 63 per cent of walkers enjoy action movies. Or 22 per cent of walkers over the age of 50 with one-legged dogs enjoy documentaries. Once these relationships have been uncovered you can use these to refine similarity searches. And here, the way dating services incorporate this into their calculations is extremely dependent on the specifics of the problem. Like how many people own one-legged dogs.

But I have made my case. Building similarity searches can be an intense exercise. A single academic might dedicate their entire life to finding ways to do this. This is not child's play! And there are still a couple of extra sticky points dating services have to incorporate into their mathematics. First, their mathematics has to be able to withstand the continually changing nature of the database that goes with people leaving and joining them regularly. Second, they have to decide when a two-way match is reached. Someone may be my closest match but whether I am theirs is another matter. Put another way, there's only one Tom Cruise and we can't all have him! The dating service is going to have to settle on some level of mutual similarity they are happy with.

And after all this, whether dating services escape the dreaded curse of dimensionality remains to be shown. But in a way that is the beauty of it. The hairy mathematics dating services face adds back the element of the unknown. From all the statistics, complicated formulae, curses, and possible meanings of similarlity, out pops a name for you. You could call this fate. Dating services provide us with the science we desire but without robbing us of our romantic ideal of 'the one that was meant to be'. What more could we want?

So similar, so what?

For dating services, people matching is about finding that special person with answers, scores or numbers most similar to yours. For mathematicians, who see everyone's numbers as a point in higher dimensional space, this translates into finding which point in space is closest to yours. At the very foundation of all the research, including the curse of dimensionality, is the pure mathematics area of higher dimensional linear algebra. Let that drop at your next barbecue. 'No, I'm not online dating anymore, I'm dabbling in a spot of pure mathematics.' It is bound to impress!

The seeds of this pure mathematics idea can be traced back to a number of mathematical thinkers from the early 19th century onwards. The main player though was the now famous Prussian-born mathematician Hermann Grassmann. The whole field of higher dimensional linear algebra seems to have blossomed when he published a couple of books around the middle of that century. Today, only a little over a century later, I doubt if a single mathematician can claim never to have dedicated part of their thinking lives to the topic.

Now, while physicists pretty much pounced on his new mathematical ideas, somehow that didn't bring much recognition to Hermann. He had a challenging intellectual life, spending much of his time as a schoolteacher desperately seeking a university position and never able to secure one. By his early fifties he had become so disappointed with this lack of interest, he basically gave up on mathematics and turned to studying Sanskrit. I am told his Sanskrit dictionary is still used today and is very good, should you ever need one.

So I would love to see Hermann's face, and all the faces of those that knew of him for that matter, if you told him his ideas would be required for the functioning of a large part of today's society, from engineering right down to 'lover-finding' at dating services.

For me this is one of the breath-taking sides of mathematics: that which might appear as the most abstract, brain-stretching, obscure notion, ends up being crucial to something unthought of and incredibly practical on a daily basis. I have come across this so many times. It really teaches you to never dismiss any idea as being useless—you just never know. Sometimes it takes thousands of years before an idea has matured enough for it to be used to its full potential. Well, maybe the idea has to wait for us to mature to fully appreciate it. Either way, original thought is one of the most beautiful aspects of being human and must be appreciated, no matter what it is. That's more for your next barbecue chit-chat.

So higher dimensional linear algebra has a lot to answer for. And the particular branch concerning dating services is in crucial development, including the curse of dimensionality. There is some big business on the horizon and it all boils down to the concept of 'similarity' as opposed to 'equality'. Until recently, the mathematics driving computers was based on the idea of 'equality'. You know what it's like when you don't type something exactly right. Your computer just returns an error message. It doesn't understand. Well, now research has turned to finding ways for a computer to respond to 'similarity'. And the idea extends way beyond recognising typos.

Information databanks are becoming larger and larger. These are useless if we can't query them properly. Say I have over a million pictures in a database, and I want to find a picture of a man with a six-pack frolicking around in the ocean. What the computer retrieves for me will depend on how the pictures have been stored or organised. If a bunch of pictures have been classified with the descriptors: 'man', 'six-pack', 'playing', 'ocean', it's my lucky day, but more than likely I will have been too specific. Six-pack might not have been catered for, maybe 'good-looking' or 'supermodel' or 'Latino' . . .

To build more effective computers, we need to get on top of the idea of 'similarity' and this by default includes the dreaded curse. And the same ideas used to locate pictures in databases more effectively are used to search for fingerprints, DNA matches, and also audio and video clips. The applications are endless.

Doesn't all junk email look similar? Being able to test incoming email for such similarities is a key to building highly efficient programs to sort out the junk from your inbox. Then there's video transmission over the Internet. That is in desperate need for a speed boost. One option being looked at is to only transmit the specific parts of each frame that aren't similar in the next one. Then there are some more commercial applications to people matching. Imagine if an airline could match people up for more enjoyable seating arrangements on flights. That's one avenue being explored, and personally I think that's a great idea! 'Yes. I'll have an aisle seat, a vegetarian meal, and a six-packed Latino with a passion for water sports.'

And then there's also love. Maybe in the future when we know a lot more about 'similarity' and the curse, we will be able to set ourselves up on the Internet and generate a bucket load of possible love-matches. I can foresee some top-quality dating on the horizon. You see, 'similarity' matching is never going to be perfect. For one, people don't describe themselves a hundred per cent accurately. Not necessarily for deceitful reasons, but because it is simply hard to be completely aware of yourself. Let's face it, that's why self-improvement gurus get so rich organising entire weekends dedicated to inner discovery. However, 'similarity' matching will still be able to help us avoid a large part of wasteful dating. So here is my vision. We'll hop on the Internet, generate a hundred or so matches as close to perfect as we can get them, then we'll date the first twelve as a test and pick the best we hook up with after that. What do you think?

$$\partial x \,/\, \partial x + \partial x \,/\, \partial x + \partial x \,/\, \partial x + \partial x \,/\, \partial x + \partial x \,/\, \partial x + \partial x \,/\, \partial x + \partial x \,/\, \partial x$$

Back to reality though: Did I find true love on the Internet? No. But I gained a lot out of the experience. I learned a lot about myself as I was forced to make a clear list of what I was after in a partner; I discovered what it feels like to routinely be the one who makes the first approach; and I met a few weirdos. I think it was all those lists of beliefs, preferences, achievements and goals that got me. Putting my entire soul on the table in one go like that was the hardest. But just because I'm hopeless at it, doesn't mean it is not an option that shouldn't be thoroughly embraced. In fact, with the way our society is going, some believe it is the way of the future. Richard Bulcroft from the University of British Columbia and Kris Bulcroft, Karen Bradley and Carl Simpson from Western Washington University have researched just why this is so. Not so long ago, our romantic decisions had a different feel. Religion and social class played much larger roles. When it came to finding a partner, many chose to marry people they knew well or entered arranged marriages. People had more than likely grown up in the same village as their future partners, had worked along side them for years, or spent considerable time with them at religious or community group gatherings. It was also natural to employ siblings, close friends, or well-known matchmakers like the parish priest, to find a suitor. Marriage was a way to gain status, join resources, become business partners or improve one's standard of living.

Today, not only do we place a huge value on individual identity, which we partially gain through love, relationships and marriage, but there has also been a near complete breakdown of socially regulated mate selection and the possibilities for marriage have expanded out of bounds. For many of us it is our personal responsibility to find a partner for which we alone wear the consequences. And we can marry someone the other side of the world of any age, religion, race, or even gender. Added to this, we also want *that* person who is going to fulfil us from A to Z and for whom we feel that enthralling all-encompassing passionate love I spoke about in the first chapter. The risks involved in love, relationships and marriage are greater than they ever have been so it is no wonder dating services have proven so popular.

And with the advancement of mathematics, the better dating services will become. But is it beginning to feel like we have been treating dating a bit too much like executing a company takeover strategy? Don't worry, there's a crucial aspect of the process, somewhat neglected in the discussions thus far, that can add a bit of a twist. There's another person involved in the equation and their say in the matter is somewhat pivotal! Next chapter . . .

Chapter 5

PAIRING UP

Remember your early teen years and those first mixed-sex parties? Talk about flirting with training wheels—full of awkward moments but at the same time very exciting. Boys and girls experiencing puberty try to look as grown up and as funky as possible—a contradiction that never quite works. The girls play shy but always manage to burst out to get the dancing happening. And the boys? Well, they like the contact of the dancing to practise their pick-up moves. Numerous phone calls the night before have probably organised who likes who anyway. And so if all goes well, targets are locked on to and the rest of the afternoon is, well, teenage bliss. Otherwise, minor reshuffle, second favourites are approached, and any rejects reshuffle again. And so the process goes on until everyone is matched, except for a few who get left aside ... as I was many times. But that's OK, I've now blossomed into a mathematician writing about mathematics and sex . . . not frustrated at all . . . nope, not at all . . .

Teenagers would probably have a fit if they found out this is actually a highly mathematical situation. Can you see mathematics? Here's a hint. Could everyone's preferences be such that no one can end up settling because someone better always seems to become available, and so the party becomes one big permanent reshuffle? (And, no, I'm not getting confused with a swinger's party.) If there's a real cutie in the group, only one person can land the babe, so how dissatisfied are the others going to be? Are there ways to increase one's chances of landing the best of the bunch? All these are questions mathematics can answer. A large part of the mathematics is very accessible to teenagers too, so I'm not quite sure why we don't teach it at school.

Now, I don't want you to go off and think there are weirdo mathematicians specialising in teenage parties. This is part of the mathematics of *game theory*. You might have already come across some of the ideas in this area, because this was the favourite mathematics of John Nash, the character Russell Crowe played in the movie, *A Beautiful Mind*. Game theory is all about strategies and outcomes in situations where different parties interact as they strive for goals. Mathematicians use it to plan corporate takeovers, political campaigns, even wars. But we are going to stick with the part of it concerned with pairing-up. And this is a problem of matching preferences.

One of the tricks of the mathematics trade is to first strip back a problem to its bare essentials to see what patterns can be uncovered. Then one can start to build in the complications. And it is often the case that the simplified version reveals a number of patterns inherent within the problem itself. This is why I mention sweet and innocent teenage party flirting. Now, I must admit I haven't been a partying teenager for a while, and my above description may be slightly out of date, but in this flirting situation, romantic decisions are pretty straightforward and one's preferences are frighteningly clear. The problem is simple: 'Are they wearing the latest?' 'No—NEEEEXT!' It's important to pair up. We want to test our choices and romance skills. And this flirting game is primary to our being. Even if our methods of classification develop to be slightly more sophisticated, and our romantic decisions to be slightly more complicated, the basics remain. What goes on in those early years is just a small-scale simplified version of what happens later in bars, among all the people we know, even across the community. Whether at a party, barbecue or among a group of friends, we have preferences and some people act on them, others sit back and wait. In fact, walking into a bar can often feel like initiating a burst of high-performance computing. You get checked out, appraised, and then allocated a position on a number of preference lists for the night. So, let me stay at the party level for the moment and ask: When Cindi Crawford or Brad Pitt appears at the gathering we're at, how far can we expect our position to drop and are there ways to soften the fall?

To make any sense of all this, it's worth simplifying the problem further. So much so, I may as well indulge in a fantasy. Say by some freak of nature, Tom Cruise, Will Smith, Hugh Grant, and Gérard Depardieu wash up on an island with four of their biggest fans: Lisa, Susan, Deborah and Queen Elizabeth II. There are only eight of them on the island. And so before too long, some pairing-up is going to happen. Who is going to end up with whom?

Here are their preferences:

Tom's preference list: Lisa, Susan, Deborah, QE II.
Will's preference list: Lisa, Susan, QE II, Deborah.
Hugh's preference list: Lisa, Deborah, QE II, Susan.
Gérard's preference list: Susan, Deborah, Lisa, QE II.

Lisa's preference list: Gérard, Tom, Will, Hugh.
Susan's preference list: Will, Gérard, Tom, Hugh.
Deborah's preference list: Will, Tom, Gérard, Hugh.
QE II's preference list: Will, Tom, Gérard, Hugh.

Since the guys are the stars, the women don't dare make any first moves. The guys make the approaches, and the women either accept or reject them. How is this going to work?

Hugh is everyone's last choice: he must be the kind of guy you marry, not the type you choose to have some fun with on an island. Who will luck out on this last straw? Lisa, as you can see, is a bit of a favourite. There is no TV on the island and her conversation has them all riveted. Tom, Will and Hugh have her in first place. Out of these three, Tom is her preferred choice, so you might expect her to pair up with him, but then he isn't her first choice, Gérard is. He's an excellent conversationalist too and that French accent is a killer. Unfortunately for Lisa though, Gérard's first choice is Susan, so Lisa might just have to settle for second best. What is going to happen? Is one person always going to feel hard done by? Can it be done so at the very least couples are never tempted to stray?

The answer to the last question is perhaps an unexpected 'yes'. Matches exist where no two people would rather abandon their respective relationships to form a new partnership together. And back in 1962 David Gale working at Berkeley and Lloyd Shapley at UCLA joined forces to show a straightforward matching method always leads to such a settled situation. Our stranded islanders happen to follow this matching method. Here's how it goes . . .

To start, the men make advances to the favourites on their lists:

Tom, Will, and Hugh, hit on Lisa.
Gérard hits on Susan.

Not knowing what's round the corner and not wanting to end up a loner on the island, Susan responds positively to Gérard's advances even though he isn't her first choice. Lisa picks the best out of her offers, and so spends some quality time with Tom. Deborah and QE II have no choice but to retire to the shade of a palm tree and eat coconuts. The conversation is polite and dignified but somewhat stilted. QE II is unhappy of course, being unfamiliar with rejection. Meanwhile . . .

Will and Hugh, rejected, shoot for the next best on their list.
Will hits on Susan.
Hugh hits on Deborah.

Susan might be with Gérard, but she prefers Will. In a flash she dumps Gérard and runs off to another corner of the island with Will. Deborah hangs out with Hugh: he might be straight-laced, but better him than another round in the lonely hearts' corner with QE II and the coconuts. For her part, QE II is now seriously annoyed but short of multiple beheadings she can see no way out of her dilemma.

Gérard, now single again, shoots for his next favourite, Deborah.

Deborah prefers Gérard to Hugh, so she dumps Hugh.

Hugh, rejected a second time, bites the bullet and shoots for his next favourite, QE II.

QE II accepts with a sigh of relief.

Final verdict: Lisa is shacked up with Tom, Susan with Will, Deborah with Gérard, and Queen Elizabeth II with Hugh.

Believe me, overall the gang is happy. Tom wouldn't want to budge as he is with his first choice. Will, Hugh and Gérard get the best they can, considering the situation. No one is tempted to stray because the ones they missed out on didn't miss out on them in return. This balanced situation might seem trivial, but believe me it's not. Change the problem slightly and overall happiness could never be on the cards. For example, pop the stars and fans together into a single group. And then try to organise general pairs to go off food gathering, by again considering lists of preferences from everyone. In this situation it may be impossible to reach a balanced situation where everyone is happy.

But with two groups to match up, there is always a final 'happy' pairing. In fact, there is more than one. We only found the one above because we used a particular matching method or technique to get it. And the larger the groups of people you're dealing with, the more possibilities there are and the more technique is important because the pairing process quickly becomes very painful without one. At a party of sixteen men and sixteen women, some preference lists can lead to over 100 000 different 'happy' pairings. So finding which one suits best is a nice thought. We can begin to extrapolate from our simplifications. Groups of people with preferences in the midst of matching themselves up. That's what our world is made of, is it not? Wouldn't it be great to know if we were in the running to score Cindi or Brad or Hugh? And if not, how far off we are?

To distinguish between pairings we look at satisfaction levels. A person's satisfaction with a pairing can be measured without too much trouble. You just look at how far down their list they had to go to reach their final partner. The further down the list, the lower the satisfaction. Adding up everyone's final partner rankings within each group then gives a measure of overall satisfaction for each group. Male and female perspectives on the final outcome can be different. In our example, the guys reach a group satisfaction level of 8, their loyal fans a level of 10. The lower the number, the better, because the number comes from rankings. So the men, even with Hugh, do better overall than the women.

But, overall group 'happiness' levels have nothing to do with how each individual feels. What if Lisa shacks up with Tom, Susan with Gérard, Deborah with Hugh, and QE II with Will? Here, the guys reach a satisfaction level of 7, the fans a level of 9. So *overall* everyone feels more satisfied than before. The problem is Will and Susan don't. And they would rather be together than the person with whom they're paired. This is sure to create unrest on the island. Group satisfaction goes out the window. What takes centre stage here is the tension between people's desires and real options.

So what is another possible pairing for our stranded islanders? One stems from turning the tables around and asking the fans to make the advances and the guys to be the accepter-rejecters. When the match is performed this way round, with the same preference lists, surprisingly another match results. This will mean, Lisa shacks up with Gérard, Susan with Will, Deborah with Tom, and QE II, well she still can't escape Hugh. And again, this is a match that sticks. Everyone lands the best partner they can. But when paired this way round, the fans are more satisfied than the guys—they reach a level of 8 and the stars reach a level of 11. And in 1997 a thorough mathematical investigation by Marie-José Oméro, Michael Dzierzawa, Matteo Marsili and Yi-Cheng Zhang, a group centred in Switzerland at the time, showed whoever proposes is always better off overall—no matter how many people there are and how big the island is. Isn't this a little counterintuitive? The ones that sit back and get to enjoy picking and choosing from a parade of potential mates are worse off in the end than the ones that painstakingly suffer through untold rejections as they move down their list to reach a match. Well, having shown the proposer's satisfaction levels obey this formula:

$$\varepsilon_H(\mathsf{M}_H) = \sum_{k=1}^{N} \frac{1}{k} \approx \log N + 0.5772 \,.$$

And the accepter-rejecter's satisfaction levels obey this formula:

$$\varepsilon_F(\mathsf{M}_H) \approx \frac{N}{\log N + 0.5772} \,.$$

It's obvious, isn't it?

What this also shows is that the more people there are to match up, the wider the gap becomes between each group's satisfaction levels. So stop hanging around the bar! Get out there and start throwing some tacky lines. Tell them you're doing it for mathematical reasons not because you're desperate. What better incentive do you want?

> Excuse me, I've been really into mathematics lately, and I can take you to infinity whenever you're ready, baby.

Mmm, I think you can see why I've never done so well at that game. But with this mathematical insight, I'm determined to keep practising. I'm not going to miss out. Yet there is one other thing. Don't run to your favourite bar just yet, there's a small complication you should be aware of: Cindi and Brad, or in other words, very attractive people!

In 2001, Italians Guido Caldarelli and Andrea Capocci found that good-lookers just skew everything. You see, in the simple 'stars and fans' island problem or in the analysis done by the Switzerland-based group, the lists were constructed at random. As if names had been put in a bag and the men and women lucky-dipped to construct their list. This means when competing for a particular spot on someone's list, everyone is equally likely to get it. But let's be realistic here, there's always a bunch of favourites that grab all the attention. And that's not random anymore. Add that to the mathematics and a different picture emerges.

Guido Caldarelli and Andrea Capocci incorporated the lack of randomness in a clever way. They saw attractiveness, or lack of it for that matter, as reflecting common opinion across lists. Their mathematical methods let you see what happens to people's satisfaction levels when common opinion grows stronger. It's as if they placed a volume dial on the attractiveness factor. When the volume is set to zero, everyone is equally likely to be picked for a particular spot on a list. We're back on our imaginary island. A set-up where the proposers do better in the end than the accepter-rejecters, and where Guido and Andrea also found that no matter which of the possible final matches people end up in, they'll always reach about the same level of satisfaction. However, if we turn up the volume by adding attractive people to the picture, they start to hog many of the people's top places on their lists and satisfaction levels no longer obey the above Oméro-Dzierzawa-Marsili-Zhang equations. Once people begin to be ranked similarly by everyone, the difference in final satisfaction levels between the proposers and accepter-rejecters starts to disappear.

With a small level of common opinion, the very attractive people whether proposers or accepter-rejecters reach similar satisfaction levels. Although, as people are deemed less attractive, the gap between proposer and accepter-rejecter satisfaction levels creeps back in, and the really unattractive accepter-rejecters fare much worse than before. But as the level of common opinion increases, or as people agree further on how desirable or not someone is, the gap closes—proposers and accepter-rejecters begin to reach similar satisfaction levels no matter how attractive or not they are. And the higher the level of common opinion, the more they do. But does the gap in satisfaction levels close because the accepter-rejecters become more satisfied or the proposers less satisfied? The proposers less satisfied, I'm afraid. But at least it's about even for both parties. At the end of the day, everyone ends up matched with someone who'll be compromising just as much as they are. And overall Guido and Andrea also found the more common opinion there is about who is attractive or not in a community, the less satisfied the community is in general. It is interesting isn't it? We find solace for our loneliness in common opinion yet the end result is less happiness. Mmm, I need to meditate on that for a while. And maybe stay away from fan-driven glossy magazines.

On a chirpier note, here is my pick-up advice (which is a scary thought, considering I couldn't even pick up at dating services!). You know on those nights when you are in a good mood, everyone is laughing at your jokes and you seem to be glowing. Those are the nights where you should sit back, relax and be funny and let the offers flow to you. At the end of the night you'll be no worse off for it. And keep telling yourself that as you stare at the phone number of the one who bored you to death all night.

However, when you find yourself at a 'beautiful people' party and you are feeling insecure, that's the time to break out. Finding out how much attention these beautiful people are actually commanding is too hard, so you may as well do something. More than likely your insecurities are taking over and you are overestimating their influence anyway. So go for it and work the room as hard as you can! If anything, I'm sure you'll have some good stories to tell your friends the next day. No matter what happens, it's 'a smile on your face'—guaranteed!

$$\partial x \, / \, \partial x + \partial x \, / \, \partial x + \partial x \, / \, \partial x + \partial x \, / \, \partial x + \partial x \, / \, \partial x + \partial x \, / \, \partial x + \partial x \, / \, \partial x$$

Forget for a second about being matched up or picking-up at a bar. Matching is pervasive in our lives. When you go for a job, you are amid a matching problem between employees and employers. Buying a car, bidding at an auction for a house, looking for a flatmate, applying for college, the list of competitive matching goes on. And the mathematics founded by Gale and Shapley in the '60s is explicitly used in a number of these types of situations. Some employment agencies indeed use it to match up employees and employers. Some economists use it to build models of society where the interaction between firms and consumers is interpreted as a matching process. It's even used by some physicists to understand the pairing up of subatomic particles. Though the most famous use of Gale and Shapley's mathematics must be in the US's National Resident Matching Program, a service that organises training placements for medical students. On average 20 000 students a year find their host hospital with this service. And whenever you consider a variety of options and make a list of preferences from which to choose from, you're becoming involved in the same mathematics too.

It is no wonder that since the '60s this problem has been considered from a whole host of perspectives. There's a whole library of mathematical analyses on the topic. What if new people come onto the scene? What if preference lists change halfway through the process? What if some people would rather stay single than pair up with what is on offer? What are the ways to manipulate the system so you can score someone better than you really are entitled to? Stop right there. This sounds like an exciting prospect. I rushed to the library to unearth the research papers. There I found that mathematics says it is impossible to design a matching technique that can never be manipulated to someone's advantage. Then there are a few pointers such as: if proposers find themselves in the situation where they are sure about everyone's preference lists, then they should never try to manipulate the system; they are better off just being honest about who they're after. But I'm not sure how helpful that is. There also are theories put forward about how to form coalitions with other people. If one person is willing to sacrifice themselves for the sake of the group, the matching process can be readily biased in someone's favour. There are recent examples of this in the 'Survivor' television series, where you can see alliances distorting who wins. There is probably a terrific mathematical paper in that series and someone out there should do it. But, back to the topic. So far, most of the findings of this research depend heavily on awareness of preferences. It's probably best then to scrap the idea of being the slick mathematical manipulator and go for preferences as you see them.

But the fact that these ideas are being so actively researched is a good sign for mathematical manipulators to come. Studying highly artificial set-ups is the start. And it is quite possible they may even reveal general patterns that we can use. Like how we now know it is better to be the one that propositions than to be the one that gracefully awaits some of the action. And there is a recent trend in academic articles to deal with incomplete information and how this affects our strategies and outcomes.

Here is where my mind short-circuits though. We develop a theory that deals with lack of information. This increases the level of information. But the more we learn, the more we find there is to know, so this means there is even more information we don't know. I need something, but I'm not sure if it's another degree or a G&T.

Chapter 6

ACTION REACTION ATTRACTION

Who do we find attractive? Can it be quantified? You can go to a plastic surgeon to have your face and body redesigned. And then you can go to a psychiatrist or do a self-improvement course to reshape your personality. There are definite boundaries there: would you like a squarer jaw, a flatter stomach, or a startling wit? I am not about to bowl you over with body and mind measurements like these. That would be as mind numbingly boring for me, as it would be for you. Besides, measuring is not what mathematics is about. That would be like believing the alphabet is what writing is about. What turns us on is a complex science; its study has involved a number of sophisticated mathematical ideas.

So let me take you on a small journey into the realm of scientific research on attraction. Well, into the three areas of mental, facial and physical attractiveness, anyway. What have been some of the findings? How has mathematics been involved? How have findings been challenged and what new ideas have emerged from the challenges?

Like all fields of endeavour, possibilities abound. But when it comes to defining attractiveness, this should be at the forefront of our minds constantly. This is an area full of subtleties, where we really have a lot to learn. To get a sense of what we do know, it seems best to just follow the path of how we obtained that knowledge in the first place. This type of insight gives us some grasp on what it is that can so magnetically draw us to someone— even though they have a hairy back, aren't as tidy as we'd like them to be, or have a tendency to be blunt at all the wrong times. You get my point. Why try and express simplicity when there isn't any?

Similarity

Do 'birds of a feather flock together' or 'opposites attract'? Most sociology textbooks favour 'the birds with the same feathers' theory and it is true that since the '60s an extremely large body of research has pointed in that direction. Despite this, in the academic world a huge debate is raging as to whether similarity and attraction really go hand in hand. In 1992, Steve Duck and Melanie Barnes from the University of Iowa named the debate the 'inverted intellectual Titanic' because 'everyone thinks it should sink but it doesn't'. Now, it is overwhelmingly the behavioural sciences that are caught up in this mess. However, there are some mathematical roots to this debate, and it also appears its complete resolution lies in a newly budding area of mathematics.

It all started in the 1930s when a couple of studies found husbands and wives had extremely similar attitudes on all kinds of subjects like church, war and communism. And this held whether they had been married a week or ten years. Was attraction and similarity related? The idea was pursued and a major breakthrough occurred in 1965 when American psychologists Donn Byrne and Don Nelson uncovered the equation:

$$Y = 5.44X + 6.62.$$

This is the relationship they found between attraction and similarity. The equation says this: when you are chatting with someone, it is not how many topics you see eye to eye on, but the *proportion* of topics on which you do that affects attraction. The higher the proportion of similar attitudes, the greater the liking will be. So if you discuss two topics like music and food, and match up on one, you will experience the same level of attraction as if you discussed four and matched up on two. And whether you are discussing how you feel about abortion or whether you like dark chocolate is secondary. It is all about proportion or quantity of similarity, not quality. Interesting, hey? I am sure this can be used in a quest to seduce someone. The key it seems is to make sure you do a lot of agreeing. But the beauty of it is you don't have to compromise when it comes to those topics you feel passionate about. Just make sure you steer the conversation on to something trivial every so often and agree with whatever view the seducee puts forth. Easy as 1, 2, 3! (Is that a maths joke?!)

Donn Byrne's mathematics didn't stop there. His next gem was produced in the same year with Ray Rhamey:

$$Y = m\left[\frac{\sum(P \times M)}{\sum(P \times M) + \sum(N \times M)}\right] + k\,.$$

What this says is the more you approve of someone's personal attributes, whether they are ideas, actions or looks, the more they will be attracted to you. So, commenting on how yummy someone's cooking is (something personal) is going to be more favourable in terms of attraction than agreeing with their views on the latest political party (something impersonal—well, for most people). As Donn Byrne puts it, 'personal evaluations must constitute *greater magnitude of reinforcement* than do attitude statements' (Byrne 1971, p. 104). Or as I put it, flattery will get you everywhere!

These two little equations from the 1960s mark the beginning of the research and debate on the influence of similarity on attraction that has raged ever since. In 1966, American psychologists George Levinger and James Breedlove found spouses assumed a greater degree of similarity than actually existed. And it was the assumed similarity that was related to marital satisfaction, not the actual similarity. Some twenty years later, in 1986, Milton Rosenbaum from the University of Iowa added significantly to the debate, with his results showing it was in fact repulsion of dissimilar attitudes rather than attraction to similar ones that drives the level of attraction. In one of his experiments, people who said nothing were rated 14.2 per cent better than those people who expressed dissimilar attitudes. Is this linked to the adage, 'When in doubt, keep your mouth shut'? Milton Rosenbaum's proposition is that we expect attitude similarity to some extent so it doesn't really do anything for us. In 1997, working at the University of North Carolina at Charlotte, Arnie Cann, Lawrence Calhoun and Janet Banks investigated how similarity in senses of humour affects attraction. We cherish humour. You know the familiar cry, 'All I want is someone who can make me laugh.' How much can a funny joke sway someone's opinion of you? Well, they found even if a person was 90 per cent dissimilar to someone else, as long as they laughed at the other's joke, they were liked more than a person who was 90 per cent similar and didn't find the joke funny. All you need is one good joke. As far as seduction tips go, I doubt if they get any easier.

So, thousands of experiments later, all kinds of relationships have been uncovered and debated in the name of finding how similarity affects attraction. Yet we really aren't that much closer to reaching a verdict. The Titanic still hasn't sunk. Then, as if all the inconsistent evidence wasn't enough, in the 1990s Michael Sunnafrank from the University of Minnesota in Duluth once again opened a real can of worms—one that mathematicians have only properly started looking into since the '80s. It is the *association* versus *causation* argument. Michael Sunnafrank agrees that attraction and similarity are associated but whether one actually causes the other is a moot point.

Let me illustrate with the classic example of smoking and lung cancer. It is true a whole variety of studies have shown smokers are prone to lung cancer. But this really only demonstrates there is an association between smoking and lung cancer. Whether one causes the other is not a logical step. And yes this is the very issue the tobacco company lawyers have been playing hardball with for years. The argument is there could be a third ingredient responsible for both these ailments to happen concurrently. There might be a genetic predisposition that causes both cancer and the need for nicotine, for example.

The same idea applies to attraction. Could there be another factor responsible for attraction between similar people? Michael Sunnafrank suggests one possibility is that the link between similarity and attraction might stem from the somewhat segregated nature of our society. If we all hang around people of similar race, socioeconomic status or age, then it might just be part of the parcel that we end up dating someone similar. It is more of a proximity thing.

Couldn't we perform some experiments to sort this out? Let me go back to smoking and lung cancer. There are some peripheral experiments we could do, but the one to nail the issue once and for all would be something like this: acquire a large group of identical twins, divide them up into two identical groups, get them to live in utterly controlled environments, make one group smoke a pack of cigarettes a day and the other remain smoke-free and then wait sixty years. Obviously, even ethical reasons aside, the difficulties associated with this experiment are voluminous. And this is a big problem faced by the social, economical and demographical sciences. How do you draw causal relationships without being able to perform tightly controlled experiments? Instead, they have to draw conclusions from studying the set-ups already existing in nature. This is vastly different to what mostly goes on in the physical, chemical and biological sciences. If a scientist wants to know what happens when an atom is split, or acid is mixed with alcohol, or an embryo is implanted, they just go ahead and do it. You see the difference: the social, economical and demographical sciences don't have the same degree of control.

Luckily for the 'softer' sciences, mathematicians are on to the problem. Is there a way to uncover a causal relationship from large population studies, studies where you can't manipulate parts of the set-up at will? Some key players in this area are Judea Pearl from UCLA and Peter Spirtes, Clark Glymour and Richard Scheines from Carnegie Mellon University. They use diagrams to visualise cause. For example:

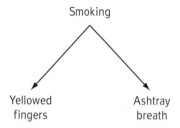

You don't have to be a mathematician to work out this means smoking causes yellowed fingers and ashtray breath. Yet a number of other things influence those three items to various degrees— like how often you lick ashtrays—and building them into the picture means the diagram quickly becomes outrageously complicated. Dealing with the complexity is one part of the problem. But, the crucial idea to understand with these diagrams is what happens if one of the items is altered. How are the other items affected? Mathematicians are setting up a whole new form of arithmetic to do that. They are working on the mathematics of *intervention* or *manipulation*.

A lot has been done, but there is still a long, long, way to go before we can say with absolute certainty that smoking causes lung cancer, similarity causes attraction or to put another idea into the mix, that divorce causes maladjusted children. This mathematics has a lot riding on it.

So, you can see, raising the issue of causation versus association in the similarity–attraction debate puts Donn Byrne and his advocates in an awkward position. It questions the logic of their arguments, but in such a way that there's no moving forward. It's like when you're having an argument and the other person says: 'Look, you're just being irrational.' It all comes to a grinding halt right then and there. You find yourself trapped. The focus of the argument has changed from the issue to the minefield that is the philosophy of logic.

So research continues. But there does appear to be an increasing tendency to search for more subtle variations in the similarity–attraction relationship. Some researchers speculate it may only be particular types of people that obey Donn Byrne's similarity–attraction equation. In 2001, Estelle Michinov and Nicolas Michinov, working at the University Blaise Pascal in France suggested a classification between high- and low-comparison oriented people. Everyone compares themselves to others from time to time. But some people go overboard. Whatever the reasons for this tendency, the Michinovs found these high-comparison oriented people seem attracted to both similar and dissimilar people. While on the other hand, their low-comparison counterparts seem to stick with only similar people, with their attraction indeed following Donn Byrne's mathematics. The idea is that high-comparison oriented people search for information about others, regardless of their similarity, to reduce the feelings of uncertainty they have about themselves.

Low-comparison people, feeling more self-assured, seek out others similar to themselves to validate their thoughts.

Similarity and attraction is clearly a multilayered problem, and we are beginning to peel away at these layers. I think we're going to see more and more of this style of research across a wide range of fields. Mathematical ideas are being used more than ever before and mathematics has an amazing capacity to unveil patterns in the most complicated of webs. But whether you are a stressed-out high-comparison person with low self-esteem or not, some scientists believe who you are attracted to will be largely governed by physical aspects anyway. So let's move on to some more superficial areas of attraction.

Facial attractiveness

Yes, I know we all have our own tastes, but it has been shown over and over again we agree remarkably well on facial attractiveness (Langlois et al. 2000). Talk politics or religion to people across the planet and an unbelievable spectrum of views will be expressed. But talk facial attractiveness and suddenly there is reasonable harmony. Something funky is going down.

Theory goes, good looks might act as predictors of mental and physical health. This makes them crucial in all forms of human interaction, especially picking up, where like peacock feathers or deer antlers, good looks act to attract and sort mates. The search is on to find exactly what facial characteristics we find attractive and how accurately they predict the state of our inner health. An interesting problem, as these characteristics would appear to be the same whether you are a Hollywood starlet or a woman from southwest Ethiopia who has stretched her lips around a plate for twenty years. Facial attractiveness goes much further than culture or fashion.

Until the 1990s the main way to conduct research in this field was to ask people to rate a catalogue of faces. Might sound fun at first, but imagine being landed with hundreds and hundreds of faces to judge. Pretty soon you'd be wishing you were scrubbing around each individual tile in the bathroom with a toothbrush, I'm sure! And yet what else can be done to get to the bottom of this? If you show people only a small quantity of faces, then the culling process involved to get this small sample in the first place is bound to skew its contents towards a particular taste. And if we are to understand how Naomi Campbell, Cameron Diaz and Goldie Hawn all fit as attractive in people's minds, we need to reflect human culture in all its variety in our sample. This is a huge job whichever way you look at it. And that's only the half of it, because once you've decided upon a top group of honeys, you then have to work out their common traits.

There is another way of looking at the problem of finding out what people deem to be attractive: getting people to build their own mega-babes from scratch. 'Hmmm, yes I think I'll have that slightly flat nose, big dark-red lips and black eyes with nicely defined eyebrows. Oh, and some long eyelashes, please. Wait, hang on, those lips are too big. Go a little smaller. Now the nose looks funny, can you make it bigger?' Here's the problem. We don't see faces as a bunch of isolated features, and trying to piece them together as a puzzle like that is fraught with difficulties. (A big issue when it comes to criminal identification, by the way.) Change the distance between the eyes, and the nose may look different; widen the mouth, and the face may seem narrower. It appears we view faces holistically. That we not only see features but also configurations. So generating a mega-babe means looking at a whole load of feature configurations or looking at all possible variations of each feature in context with all possible variations of all other features. This seems more daunting than ploughing through pages and pages of pre-prepared faces. And again bathroom cleaning is starting to look like an appealing alternative.

But the idea is not to be given up on because it has the potential to unearth other aspects of attraction. Is there a common ideal? Do people have preferences for features that are in fact plausible? Could Pamela Anderson's supernormal features and proportions really be norms of sexiness? In 1993, Victor Johnston and Melissa Franklin from New Mexico State University found a way to quickly build a babe with the mathematics of genetic algorithms. Now they didn't come up with Pamela, but I'd say her features match pretty well the preferences they found. If you can introduce me, I'll measure up her face and check for sure.

Computers are built with algorithms, which are just recipes. This is because computers work by following rules and need to be told exactly what to do in every eventuality. You take one of those, mix it with three of those, wait five seconds and there you have it. Writing a computer recipe is a highly mathematical exercise. Conjuring up all possible eventualities and working out how the computer should deal with each of them is a feat of analysis, logic and creativity.

Genetic algorithms are a particular type of algorithm or recipe, which were a neat invention from the '60s. Their distinctive characteristic is that they follow the structure of biological evolution. Natural selection, mutation and crossover have proven to be powerful tools when it comes to developing life on Earth. And the same ideas have proven to be powerful in improving computer performance. It is best illustrated in the context of an example so let me go right ahead and explain how Victor Johnston and Melissa Franklin's algorithm worked.

The algorithm was designed to help subjects build a female bombshell. Our researchers started by setting up a system that encapsulated faces, or their individual features and proportions, into one big number. Specific distances between the eyes, types and positions of foreheads, shapes of mouths etc. were all given a number. These numbers were then joined in a row to make one big number representing a particular combination of features and proportions. So let's say Cameron Diaz and Goldie Hawn share the same distance between their chin and mouths, and it is chin–mouth distance 101. And Cameron's eyes are number 0, and Goldie's number 1. Then Cameron's face number would be 1010 and Goldie's 1011. (I'm only using the digits 0 and 1 because that's what you have to do for computers.) Victor Johnston and Melissa Franklin's face numbers were slightly bigger of course. Theirs had thirty-four digits, which allows for over 17 billion different faces. Let me make Cameron and Goldie's face numbers a little bigger then to make things a little more realistic:

Cameron's:	10100011101
Goldie's:	10110100111

Can you see the genetic analogy yet? These strings can be compared to strings of DNA. Just like DNA, they are the construction plans that dictate how the face is to be built.

Victor Johnston and Melissa Franklin generated thirty random face numbers, or, in other words, thirty random faces, from which a subject could commence their bombshell search. They asked men and women to have a crack at it. Subjects began by giving each of these faces a beauty mark out of ten. The algorithm then did the following. It put the top ranking face aside and then entered the remaining twenty-nine into a raffle, with each face allocated a number of tickets based on its ranking: the higher its ranking, the more tickets it had and the more likely it was to win. The algorithm then 'bred' the raffle winner with the top-ranked face to create two new faces. What this means exactly is explained below.

Finding the top-ranked face and the raffle-winning face is the natural selection part of the genetic algorithm—two good faces are picked out, with a bit of luck mixed in because of the raffle. Their 'breeding' involves the crossover and mutation part. Again the idea is completely genetic.

Crossover has occurred to the DNA in our eggs and sperm. These sex cells are born out of standard cells that usually contain a set of DNA from our mother and a set from our father. Sex cells contain half this amount, and their making therefore involves DNA from a standard cell separating into two equal amounts. But before this happens, strands from the mother and father DNA break off and swap positions—they cross over. This appears to be a clever evolutionary strategy, because it gives the opportunity for some genetic variety. Otherwise, we would be very close to clones of our grandparents and we wouldn't stumble across new and improved traits so easily. The same idea is used in genetic algorithms.

How did Victor Johnston and Melissa Franklin's algorithm get the raffle-winning face and the top-ranked face to do some crossing over? It just swapped some of their digits around. Cameron's and Goldie's faces might experience crossover like this:

| Cameron's: | 10110011101 |
| Goldie's: | 10100100111 |

Here, I have crossed the first four digits. In the algorithm, *where* this happened was random, and *how much* was prescribed.

This is the first part of the breeding process. The next part is the mutating. Making sex cells is an extremely complicated and intricate process and this means the DNA probably won't emerge unscathed. It is quite likely the DNA will end up with a few, hopefully small, random changes. These are mistakes if you like, but shouldn't be seen negatively as they represent potential for genetic improvement. In the algorithm, mutation meant changing random digits from 0 to 1 or vice versa. How much mutation could occur was prescribed, or capped if you like, so the digits didn't end up in a complete jumble.

The end result of the breeding process: two new faces that were slight modifications of the top-ranked and raffle-winning faces. The crossovers and mutations enabled these faces to be combined, while at the same time ensuring a few new added features were explored for potential.

That's the algorithm. From here, each subject was asked to give these two new faces a beauty mark. If one of these faces received a mark higher than the bottom-ranked face from the last group, then it joined the group and the bottom-ranked face was dumped. Then the algorithm started again: the top-ranking face was put aside; the remaining twenty-nine were entered into the raffle; the winner 'bred' with the top-ranked face and two new faces were born, ready to be ranked for the opportunity to join the group. As this process was repeated over and over again, faces with the subject's preferred qualities evolved.

So how did Victor Johnston and Melissa Franklin's mathematical experiment go? Well first, the genetic algorithm approach proved to be quite efficient. Even though it contained a potential for over 17 billion different faces, on average it took appraising only seventy-seven faces to achieve the bombshell. Second, subjects felt quite confident this procedure did in fact give them the freedom to build their bombshell, to the point where some male subjects requested a copy of their final face to take home. I should also add that as a follow-up study the final faces were given to others for judgment and they were consistently picked as being more attractive and youthful out of a whole array of faces. These faces definitely had something to reveal about our female beauty preferences. The analysis: lips and lower jaws seem to do it for us. It appears we fantasise about women with shorter than average lower face measurements, fuller than average lips, and smaller than average mouth width. And the only real difference between the male and female views was women had a thing for larger lower lips. What on earth does this mean? Well, besides good news for the collagen industry.

Victor Johnston and Melissa Franklin answer this question with a sexual selection explanation. Sexual selection advocates that as part of the evolutionary process we evolved some distinct characteristics simply to attract the opposite sex. Being sexually attractive will of course make us more successful at passing on our genes. And since attracting is a two-way process, it has been proposed sexy characteristics probably didn't evolve ad hoc but were selected on the basis of potential for reproductive success. Because, evolutionarily speaking, it's that potential we are after. And for women this is thought to boil down to health and high fertility. Now since women don't have any direct cues to signal these traits, the search has been on for some more subtle indirect ones. How about fuller lips and shorter lower-face measurements?

Turns out fuller lips may stem from a surge of oestrogen at puberty. And shorter lower-face measurements from lower levels of the more masculine sex hormones at puberty. Subtle is the word if this was men's main cue for a woman's health and fertility. But this fits in nicely with one of the most acclaimed studies in support of this 'health–high-fertility sexual selection' theory: Devendra Singh's waist-to-hip ratio study. Let me explain.

Devendra Singh found men judged women with waist-to-hip ratios close to 0.7 particularly attractive, usually in the range 0.68 to 0.72. The ratio is calculated by dividing the waist measurement by the hip measurement. So Cameron Diaz, who according to www.babewarehouse.com has the measurements 34–23–32, has a waist-to-hip ratio of $23 \div 32 = 0.72$, while Pamela Anderson, with measurements 36–24–36, has a waist-to-hip ratio of $24 \div 36 = 0.67$. Since Cameron barely scrapes into the sexy range and Pamela is outside of it altogether, they must be too ugly to fit Devendra Singh's study. Hmmm . . .

Davendra Singh's sexual selection link is that waist-to-hip ratios around the 0.7 mark appear to be indicative of good health and hormonal status, and therefore fertility. Women with around about a 0.7 ratio have low incidences of type II diabetes, gallbladder disease, heart disease, strokes, and carcinomas of the endometrium, ovary and breast; they show low levels of testosterone and experience puberty a little earlier as well. Also women with a higher ratio seem to have more trouble falling pregnant.

Victor Johnston and Melissa Franklin's suggestion is that these hormonal patterns of low waist-to-hip ratio women also foster fuller lips and shorter lower face measurements. Some women just have it all: attractive faces, a body to die for, and no gallbladder disease.

The arguments are convincing. The puzzle fits together so well. Well, not quite. Let me show you where some of the mathematical analysis is wonky.

Waist-to-hip ratio

In the 1990s Devendra Singh from the University of Texas set out to test the widely held belief that definitions of sexiness change with the times. I mean we all hear about the plump women in Rubens' paintings, and Marylin Monroe's large dress-size, followed by the more modern stick-looking Twiggy and then of course Kate Moss. But are we making wild generalisations here again by saying our physical turn-ons have fluctuated like the seasons? Because if they have, something isn't quite fitting.

If physical attraction has evolved from our cave-dwelling past as a cue in sexual selection, some physical turn-ons should stay constant not only throughout the years but also cross-culturally.

As the Marylin Monroe versus Kate Moss argument suggests, studies show our icons of female beauty have indeed weighed steadily less, even had smaller and smaller breasts, so what could be staying constant? Devendra Singh turned to body-fat distribution. Men and women have marked differences in this area. In particular, men carry it easily on their stomach (think beer bellies) and women carry it easily on their bottoms and thighs (think stereotype of woman nagging her boyfriend about the look of her butt in the potential new jeans). The main reason for this difference is hormonal. Testosterone stimulates fat deposition in the gut area and fat utilisation in the butt and thigh area. Oestrogen does the opposite. (How does my oestrogen look in these jeans?) And waist-to-hip ratios have shown to be a reliable indicator of body fat distribution with women's ratios usually sitting between 0.67 and 0.8 and men's between 0.85 and 0.95.

How could Devendra Singh study how the fat distribution changed from one sexy woman to the next throughout the years? Using Playboy centrefolds and winners of the Miss America pageant, of course. Part of their job description is to have waist and hip measurements recorded for all to see. Brilliant to think what at first seems so superficial ends up being crucial scientific evidence. Devendra Singh calculated the waist-to-hip ratio for all Playboy centrefolds from 1955 to 1965 and from 1976 to 1990 (measurements from 1966 to 1975 were unavailable to him), and all Miss America winners from 1923 to 1987 (measurements were no longer recorded after 1987 because of a policy change). And out popped the magic sexy waist-to-hip ratio range 0.68 to 0.72. Nice. Even though these women did become more slender, their waist-to-hip ratio stayed about the same.

Knowing full well this study was far from conclusive on the matter, Devendra Singh performed some further experiments. All substantiated the fact that men like women with a low waist-to-hip ratio. This is such a pleasing result that it has been, and still is, quoted ad nauseam. So let me stop here and turn to the work of two sociologists from the University of Wisconsin-Madison, Jeremy Freese and Sheri Meland. They weren't a hundred per cent sold on Devendra Singh's work and needed convincing that our sexiness preferences really were governed by such precision. So they combed through the original Playboy/ Miss America study with a mathematical fine-tooth comb and happened to stumble on a bit of a tangle.

They went right back to scratch and began by regathering all the waist and hip measurements for the Playboy centrefolds and Miss America winners. Here they were able to fill in some gaps. They extended the Playboy centrefold data to include the centre-folds up to May 2001 (Singh stopped at 1990) and they found most of the Playboy centrefold data between the years 1966 to 1975 that had been excluded. They added the 1921 and 1922 Miss America winners to the data too. And through this process, they came across something interesting: a number of sources reported Miss America measurements, and the data in the one Devendra Singh used had been rounded by half-inches, sometimes it seemed arbitrarily up or down. Marilyn Buferd, Miss America 1946, had given her measurements as 35–25.5–36 to the Atlantic City newspaper, but Singh's data pool used 35–25–36.

And there were quite a few of these. Now you may think the fact they even took notice of such difference is geekily pedantic, but when it comes to ratio calculations this lack of detail can wreak havoc. Look. According to the Atlantic City newspaper Nancy's waist-to-hip ratio would be 0.71, but according to the rounded data it would be 0.69. A big difference when in the first place you're really only interested in the numbers between 0.67 and 0.8—the numbers women usually reach.

Armed with this added information, Jeremy Freese and Sheri Meland searched for the relatively constant waist-to-hip ratio, but could no longer justify it. In fact not only did the waist-to-hip ratios now range from 0.529 to 0.788 (were some of these ladies gravely ill?), but it also appeared the ratio for the Miss Americas followed a curve over the years, not a straight line. Miss America waist-to-hip ratios declined until about 1969, at which point they started to increase back up again. At the same time, the Playboy centrefold waist-to-hip ratios simply increased slightly and steadily over the years.

Maybe these clusters of sexy icons cater for specific waist-to-hip ratio fetishes? And maybe what men find sexy in general is far from precise? With their understanding of mathematics Jeremy Freese and Sheri Meland have put a touch of reality back into the fast-growing cult of waist-to-hip ratio sexiness. They have also managed to further establish Playboy as an important scientific research tool. Which is another reason for reading Playboy besides the articles.

$$\partial x \,/\, \partial x + \partial x \,/\, \partial x + \partial x \,/\, \partial x + \partial x \,/\, \partial x + \partial x \,/\, \partial x + \partial x \,/\, \partial x + \partial x \,/\, \partial x$$

There are plenty more investigations along the same lines as the ones I've just shown you, which aim to isolate characteristics of attractiveness, using mathematics to various degrees. Even if our vision is still blurred, we can begin to see vague hints of what it might be that makes someone attractive (to us?). But I think, in an unashamedly biased way, for our knowledge to soar we need to use stacks more mathematics!

Mathematics has already been used extensively in our quest to find how similarity affects attraction, and whether women with shorter than average lower face measurements, fuller than average lips, and particular waist-to-hip ratios are more attractive. But much of the research has focused on a single cause along with a single effect. The true strength in mathematics lies in tackling the problem of how numerous causes and effects are interwoven. That is why I like Jeremy Freese's and Sheri Meland's investigation of the waist-to-hip ratio so much. With a little bit of extra mathematics they embraced complexity, they stopped focusing on trying to make everything fit neatly into a single box. And I feel there has been a little too much 'box-squeezing' going on in this field.

Take bilateral symmetry as another example. Bilateral symmetry has been shown by a number of researchers to be particularly attractive (Grammer & Thornhill 1994). Draw an imaginary line down the middle of your face and if what lies on the right matches up with what lies on the left, you're a good-looking sort. This theory is particularly appealing from a social psychology point of view because symmetry appears to signal good genes and good health. Only good-quality stock is thought to be able to maintain symmetric development. And that's the only type of stock with whom we want to have sex (or with whom to pair-up with to pass on our genes). Randy Thornhill, Steven Gangestad, and Randall Comer, from the University of New Mexico, have even found women have more orgasmic sex with men with symmetric faces than asymmetric ones. But symmetry measurements only work when the person is static, and this is where the theory unravels a little. Once a person is talking and being emotive, their face far from maintains symmetry. In fact around 76 per cent of people speak with greater movement on the right side of their mouth (Burt & Perrett 1997), but when being emotive, the left side of the face is more expressive than the right. A spontaneous smile can be quite bent to the left and posed smiles have a tendency to be symmetric (Skinner & Mullen 1991), and spontaneous smiles consistently rate as being more attractive than posed ones (Kowner 1996). So you see my point. At which stage in the dating game do we get to stare at the other face-on while they are not moving or speaking to do a symmetry analysis? There is no doubt there are subtleties involved. And I think we may be searching for a simple answer where there just isn't meant to be one.

Mathematicians study all kinds of symmetries. Symmetry doesn't just have to be bilateral. There's rotational symmetry, translational symmetry, algebraic symmetry . . . Mathematicians see

$$\frac{\partial}{\partial u}\left(\frac{\partial z}{\partial v}\right) = \sin(z)$$

as symmetric, and have even found symmetries in Picasso's paintings given by (Nyikos et al. 1994):

$$N(r) \propto \tau^{-D_b}.$$

Shouldn't all symmetries be good candidates as signals of good genes and good health? We are talented at recognising all kinds of patterns. Investigating other symmetries might explain why David Bowie is still extraordinarily attractive, even though he has different coloured eyes and crooked teeth. Now if they could explain how Cher fits in the picture as well, that would be greatly appreciated.

When it comes to defining attractiveness, I'm not convinced searching for a simple and pure default position is a worthy pursuit. We are dealing with multilayered problems. Why search for a simple answer and then dangle all the subtle variations around the edges? All-encompassing theories can exist and I believe mathematics is the perfect tool to get us there.

Some people believe life is beautifully simple, I believe it is beautifully complex. Then again, I am often told to stop analysing everything so much and take things more on face value. Didn't I just say some research has found men with symmetric faces provide more orgasms? Maybe it's time I simplified my life after all.

Chapter 7

PICK A SEX, ANY SEX

Have you ever found yourself wishing there was another sex? Maybe you have secretly wished for a sex with a penis that would cry with you at the movies, or a sex with breasts that would find copious beer drinking the greatest turn-on since Elvis. Or maybe you're just into variety.

Stereotypes aside, why our choice of sexual partner is limited to one sex (or maybe two, at best!) is an interesting question. Some slime moulds can choose from among three sexes. *Stylonychia lemnae*, tiny organisms commonly found in ponds, can enjoy the variety that comes with forty-eight sexes. Certain fungi have a choice of several thousands of sexes with which to mate. And asexual organisms have no choice at all. Yet, at the end of the day, it appears nature has had a penchant for dual sexuality. This is the case right down to the most basic unicellular organisms.

But why is this and is it a stable set of affairs? We often forget we are still immersed in the evolutionary process. Could boy bands like *NSYNC be the nascent branching out of a new sex? Mathematics, I am pleased to say, has answers!

What is a sex exactly?

This does need a little clarification. 'A sex' is better referred to as 'a mating type'. In a sexually reproductive population, certain individuals will be compatible with others to form offspring, while others won't—forget about looks, nooks and appendages, it all boils down to that possibility. Denzel Washington, Sean Connery and Halle Berry all look vastly different, but when it comes to making babies, Denzel or Sean will have to sleep with Halle. We have a division into two mating types. It doesn't matter what Denzel and Sean do behind closed doors, babies ain't going to happen.

Even in sexually reproducing organisms made up of only a single cell, it is often the case that genes only allow the cells to mate with certain other unique cells. Mating types are a common theme. Which leads to the question: if more than two mating types are present in a population, who is to have sex with who? Say there were three sexes: males, females and memales. How could reproduction be set up?

Situation 1: As long as you both belong to a different sex, you will be able to reproduce. So, females would have the choice to mate with either males or memales, memales with either males or females, and then males with either females or memales.

Situation 2: Two specific sexes have to come together to reproduce. So for example, males could only mate with females, and likewise memales could only mate with females. This set-up is not counted as a possibility by many researchers because it can be seen as a version of the Denzel, Sean and Halle story. Denzel and Sean look different, like males and memales might, but they can both only produce offspring by mating with the one other sex Halle, or females. We have Denzel and Sean or males and memales in one group, and Halle or females in the other. It really amounts to a two-sex set-up.

Situation 3: Two sexes need each other for reproduction, but one sex reproduces asexually. Which sex would you like to belong to in this case?

Situation 4: All three sexes need to come together at once to reproduce. A threesome every time! Might sound exciting to some, but this situation has never been found in the wild and the logistics of it ever existing have been discarded. It is not hard to see why evolution has not gone down that path. Just think of how hard it is already to pick up in our set-up. Imagine if you had to pick up two people each time. You would hardly ever get laid and the population would die out faster than you could say 'your place or mine?'

OK. That deals with three sexes. Say there were four sexes: males, females, memales and vemales.

Situation 1: Males and females can reproduce. Memales and vemales can reproduce.

Situation 2: Males and females can reproduce. Memales and vemales can reproduce. Females and memales can reproduce.

Situation 3: . . .

Aaaaaah. How tedious is this?! There has to be a better way to get a grasp of such ideas without painstakingly going through every step. What if you want to understand the choices of a mushroom with mating types in the tens of thousands? Mathematics to the rescue. Mathematics can bring simplicity to what appears at first glance to be mind-boggling.

In the late '80s, researchers James Bull and Craig Pease from the University of Texas realised this problem is one of combinatorics and graph theory. Combinatorics—you can see the connection with 'combinations'—is the study of all possible enumerations, combinations and permutations you can perform within a group of objects. Graph theory comes in handy here because it is a way to visualise the different combinations. Each mating type is represented by a dot. And if two mating types can produce offspring, the dots are joined by a line. Here are the graphs James Bull and Craig Pease studied as representations of how a population made up of three sexes could be organised into reproductive sexual partners:

And here are those they studied for how a population made up of four sexes could be organised:

The beauty is there are a whole host of theorems and formulae set up in graph theory, a field that has been flourishing since the 1930s. From them you can tell straight off the bat that, for example, there are five possible ways a population of four mating types could be organised (see second diagram above), there are 588 ways a population of seven mating types could be organised, and 10 014 882 ways a population of ten mating types could be organised.

Now I know we could all keep dinner party guests riveted by rattling off such numbers, but there is actually more to it than that. It turns out organisms with more than one sex don't embrace this possible structural variety. There has definitely been a preference for the structure where each sex can have sex with any other sex to reproduce. That means organisms favour the graph with all the dots joined by lines to all other dots—these are the graphs on the far right in both of the above diagrams. Out of all the graphs that could describe their reproductive set-up organisms prefer this unique situation. And the numbers enable us to appreciate to what degree—organisms with ten mating types, for example, forgo 10 014 881 sexual set-ups for this one structure. This just can't be by fluke.

Now at first you might think: 'Yeah, that's obvious. That gives more choice, more chance of having sex, more chance of reproduction. Sure, I'd go for that.' And it is true the prevailing theory is just that. But if nature lends itself to making sure we have a good chance of reproduction, why are populations with only two sexes favoured? Out of all the possible numbers, it turns out that two sexes gives the worst odds of finding a partner. Just think. If there were no sexes, then finding a partner is not an issue. If there were three sexes, then you could choose between two-thirds of the total population; four sexes, between three-quarters of the population. If there were a hundred sexes, you could choose between the other 99 per cent. The more sexes, the higher your chance of getting laid. Well, this assumes the number of individuals in each sex category is roughly equal, but that usually happens anyway—another story. You can see how in a population of two sexes, you're going to be left with only being able to choose a partner from half the total population—the situation with the worst odds of getting laid. That just has to be the best excuse for those long single patches most of us find ourselves in from time to time, don't you think? How on earth did we end up this way?

There are two major theories: one is based on population dynamics, the other on cytoplasmic parasitic genes. Sounds impressive?

Population dynamics

Population dynamics is the mathematical study of how populations develop and distribute themselves over time. A study might concern population size, age distribution or how a particular trait, like hairy ears, spreads. So let's say by some freaky mutation, instead of the proverbial two heads, you ended up with a third sex. Could the third sex spread throughout the initially bisexual population? And how would it?

Japanese scientists Yoh Iwasa and Akira Sasaki from Kyushu University in Fukuoka realised this had to be analysed at the level of chromosomes where sex is determined. In humans, two of our forty-six chromosomes are sex-chromosomes. They are referred to as X and Y. Women usually have two Xs (XX), men one X and one Y (XY). What would happen if a third sex-chromosome, Z, was among the population?

Yoh Iwasa and Akira Sasaki considered the sex determination pattern of a generic trisexual population as:

Females: XX
Males: XY, YY
Memales: XZ, YZ, ZZ

Here, any organism with a Z chromosome is part of the third sex. Note the YY possibility. In our set-up where we have only females and males, it doesn't exist. But Yoh Iwasa and Akira Sasaki are broadening horizons to study other set-ups, so all possibilities must be considered. This is not just some fancy intellectual exercise. Some single-celled organisms are 'sexually set-up' this way and it has been viewed as one of the most likely scenarios. The theory of evolution suggests life on Earth began with no sexes and that some life forms then developed two, then some three and so on. Did our sexuality just stop at two or did we go to a higher number and then come back down to two? And in either case, why? Could this trisexual set-up have been a phase we and most other organisms went through at the dawn of animal existence some thousand million years ago? The answers lie in using population dynamics to see how such a trisexual population would evolve. Yoh Iwasa and Akira Sasaki analysed how a Z chromosome would spread in a previously Z-free population.

With the population sorted into sex-chromosome carriers, an analysis of reproduction patterns may begin. We'll consider the case where any two different sexes can reproduce together.

Say for example, a male XY and a memale XZ reproduce. This couple will be equally likely to make a female XX, a male XY, or memales XZ or YZ. So two times out of four they are likely to have a memale even though their genetic make-up may be different. If they have a female XX and she reproduces with an YZ memale, the original couple can expect to have either XY males or XZ memales as grandchildren. But if they have an XZ memale and it (he? she?) reproduces with an XY male, their options for grandchildren are larger. They can expect XX females, XY males, XZ memales or ZY memales. Confusing? Stay with me.

A huge chain of events unfolds. The type of children the original couple have affects what type of grandchildren to expect, what type of great grandchildren, and great great grandchildren, and on it goes. Look at this for all the types of females, males and memales, and it begs the question of what type of sexual split will have emerged in the population in some future generation. Will there be equal numbers of all three sexes? Maybe only two of the sexes will flourish, while the other struggles to keep its numbers? We are in the midst of population dynamics. And the Japanese scientists worked out this population unfolding is much better understood with

$$F_{11}' = M_{12}p/2 + M_{13}q/2 + M_{23}pq/4\,,$$

$$F_{12}' = M_{12}[p/2 + (1-p)] + M_{13}(1-q)/2$$
$$+ M_{23}[pq/4 + p(1-q)/4 + (1-p)q/2]\,,$$

$$F_{22}' = M_{23}[p(1-q)/4 + (1-p)(1-q)/2]\,,$$

$$F'_{13} = M_{13} / 2 + M_{23} p / 4 \,,$$

$$F'_{23} = M_{23}[pq / 4 + p(1 - q) / 4 + (1 - p)q / 2 + (1 - p)(1 - q) / 2] \,,$$

$$F'_{33} = 0 \,,$$

topped off with a hit of 'mating kinetics'. Yeah, right!

What mating kinetics sounds like to some, like me, and what it actually means might be different. It actually refers to your *opportunities* for sexual intercourse (not possible motions during). In our trisexual population each sex has the option to have sex with two other sexes. And the more sexually mature organisms there are in each sex, the more likely you are of producing offspring with them. There is strength in numbers. The complication is the numbers are continually changing. They depend on which types of organisms got together in the previous generation, which types they had as offspring, the time lag before organisms reach sexual maturity, and how long organisms live for or are able to give offspring production a go. These 'mating kinetics' factors are a key to working out how the number of organisms in each sex changes over the generations. And it is all in the equations. And doing the mathematics will lead to a description of the future sexual split. The mathematics acts like cranking a handle on a time machine.

So what destiny do the equations predict for a Z chromosome emerging from nowhere? Should Z chromosome carriers invest in trust funds for their heirs, or won't they have any and so shouldn't worry? Here is the story the equations tell.

First, assuming the Z chromosome is not rubbishy, it and its host enjoy some privileges. As a rare sex, it will basically be able to have sex with anything and everything in sight, and produce offspring or spread its sex chromosome like wild fire. Until of course it isn't so rare! (Like Australian actors in Hollywood, the novelty has to wear off eventually.) For a brief moment in time, the three sexes might coexist in harmony. Yet the equations are clear: there won't be a perfect balance and one of the sexes is going to be driven to extinction. But here is the twist: it doesn't have to be the Z chromosome that goes. If Z has anything worthy on it, it could quite easily gain a strong hold on the population and engender a sex turnover! Yep, that's right. Either the X or Y can get pushed out of the way.

Mathematics reveals basic evolutionary processes lead to a prevalent return to dual sexuality. Population morphology can also change because of standard genetic variations. This could also be added to the mix, but it isn't needed. By simply studying who can reproduce with who at each generation, you find that populations prefer having two sexes. The equations show that it is only really when there is a significant cost associated with waiting to have offspring that many sexes have the opportunity to establish themselves. Fungi, with sexes in the thousands, might fit into this category. They are immobile and have no choice but to be a little more patient when it comes to finding a compatible mate. It could very well be that this wait involves costs leading to it being advantageous to have more sexes than you can poke a stick at.

So according to Yoh Iwasa and Akira Sasaki our very distant relatives could quite conceivably have had to deal with third sex invasions. They may have been rare but the researchers are keen with their strong mathematical results for us to investigate the matter of sexuality further. Traces of such disruption are sure to exist. If we classified sexes more carefully, might we uncover more organisms with three of more sexes? The honeybee is an interesting mix. Populations consist of females or queens; sterile males or drones; and another group of males, the workers, who are fertile and genetically very distinct as they possess only half the number of chromosomes as the other two.

And what about the future: is it likely memales might develop sometime and wipe either males or females out? Well, it is not beyond the realm of the imagination and you just never know what nature has in store. But let's hope these memales like to put the toilet seat down because with the Y chromosome in the state it is in, it doesn't look like the X chromosome is going anywhere soon. The Y chromosome in males has evolved to be very small and not to carry very much information. We need an X to function properly. When nature has got itself in a bit of a knot, people have been born all kinds of ways: with one X, two Xs and a Y, or two Ys and a X. But never have we seen someone with only one Y or two Ys. So, if a sex chromosome has to go, it's bound to be the Y. Then again, if we are willing to fantasise about time travel, world peace and the appearance of memales, why not also entertain the possibility that one day the Y chromosome will wiggle itself into a more necessary position and so won't go . . . So many possibilities!

Before we let our imaginations run too wild though, there is another theory that points to the strength in having two sexes. It is the cytoplasmic parasitic gene theory and it doesn't lend itself to the potential for so much upheaval.

Cytoplasmic parasitic genes

Before we hit the mathematics, we need a short crash course in cell biology. If nothing else, the phrase 'cytoplasmic parasitic genes' needs clarification.

All cells within multi-celled animals and plants are made of a nucleus sitting among cytoplasm, all of which is contained within a membrane. The cytoplasm is full of machinery necessary for the survival of the cell. For example, there can be mitochondria to convert foods into usable energy, ribosomes to manufacture proteins and lysosomes as sites of digestion. Our cells usually contain all three.

Both the nucleus and mitochondria contain DNA. Still, only the DNA in the nucleus makes up our genetic blueprint; that is, our chromosomes. Befittingly, cells can afford to be casual about their number of mitochondria but certainly not about their number of nuclei. Nuclei should only appear solo. In contrast, a cell may contain a couple to thousands of mitochondria. The number varies according to the amount of energy the cell needs for its duties. Your average heart muscle cell, for example, has many more mitochondria than your average skin cell.

A few characteristics differentiate nuclear DNA from mitochondrial DNA. What has captured the minds of scientists though is the number of similarities between mitochondrial DNA and bacterial DNA. One theory is mitochondria evolved from bacteria taking up residence inside other primitive cells. As if all our worst fears had come true, it appears we represent the culminating result of a codependent relationship. Everything about us goes back to how well those two little cells got on over a thousand million years ago and how they ended up needing each other for survival. And according to a group of researchers including Laurence Hurst from the University of Bath, Vivian Hutson from the University of Sheffield and Richard Law from the University of York, this holds right down to our sexuality.

When you think 'sex' you might as well think 'eggs and sperm'. These are also cells, generically referred to as gametes, with a nucleus and mitochondria, both containing DNA. The nuclei of gametes contain only half the amount of chromosomes or DNA of usual cells, so when egg and sperm join, a cell with the full amount of nuclear DNA is formed. But when it comes to the amount of mitochondrial DNA found in eggs and sperm compared to that found in other cells, there is no real difference. And here something interesting happens upon an egg–sperm join. Usually, over the course of a few days the sperm's mitochondrial DNA disappears. Sperm and egg combine the information contained in their nuclei but not that from their mitochondria. In that area, the egg has right of way. Peter Sutovsky and his colleagues working at Oregon Health Sciences University found reason to believe enzymes in the egg actively exterminate the foreign sperm mitochondrial DNA.

Let's recap a little. Eggs have evolved as complements to sperm in the nuclear DNA department, but as war initiators in the mitochondrial DNA department. It is time to pause again and realise the wonder of what is going on here. How is it we emerge so perfectly from such a conflicting mix of harmonious and contentious DNA interactions? Isn't reproduction just, as Laurence Hurst puts it, 'a marvel of communication and co-ordination' (1995)?

DNA's mission is to replicate itself. Sure, if DNA combines its strengths with those of other DNA it will increase its chances of a future existence. But the act of combination also opens the door to many events besides strength building, like contamination by defects or diseases, or development of selfish or parasitic DNA. Selfish DNA is DNA that has evolved to ensure it is preferentially transmitted through the generations, no matter what its effect, whether it be strength or weakness. Now since foreign mitochondria appear to be so vehemently disliked by eggs, and since mitochondria have their own DNA, the spotlight shines straight in their direction. Was this rejection of sperm mitochondrial DNA born from a response to selfish mitochondria behaviour? Quite possibly and, as I'm about to show, from a mathematical standpoint, the mere goal to limit this competition between different mitochondrial DNA easily accounts for why two sexes evolved from none and why more than two sexes might be more trouble than they're worth. And this fits observation nicely: fungi with sexes in the thousands, and *Stylonychia lemnae*, those tiny organisms that can be one of forty-eight sexes, both only exchange nuclear material but no cytoplasmic material when they mate. In organisms where gametes fuse but one's cytoplasmic material dominates, certain slime moulds are basically the only ones that carry more than two sexes. And even then the number of sexes mostly only escalates to three or four.

How does fighting selfish or parasitic mitochondrial activity turn into sexuality? In 1993 Vivian Hutson and Richard Law gave us a recipe for dual sexuality (which you actually may *not* like to try at home).

Recipe for dual sexuality

INGREDIENTS:

1 sexless population of organisms

1 parasite

3 mutations

PREPARATION:

Begin with a sexless population of organisms whose cells are built with nucleus and cytoplasm, and who, like us, produce gametes with half the amount of nuclear DNA. With no sexual differentiation, all gametes are quintessentially the same—no gender differences—and each organism can mate with any other. I'll spare you the details of how these organisms might seduce each other; suffice to say if they 'get into each other' and two of their gametes unite, the resulting offspring emerges with a complete set of nuclear DNA and inherits cytoplasm from both parents. Now to help out with this recipe, I've come up with an illustration: an organism with a point and a slot as sexual equipment that I couldn't help but name a 'pointy-slot'.

While I now deeply regret not having spent more time on my arty side, I think you can see without too much imagination how, in this world of one-sex, a point in a slot will produce offspring.

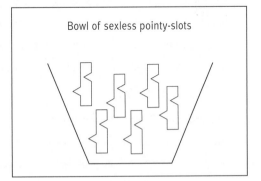

Bowl of sexless pointy-slots

STEP 1 The two-sex recipe begins in earnest when we add a cyto-plasmic parasite to the sexless mix. In the real world, this could be a bacterium, which ends up residing in some but not all organisms. To make sure this recipe works, we need the parasite to have slightly detrimental effects on its host's health. But not too much, otherwise the sexless pop-ulation could be eradicated and our recipe will have failed. Here, the para-site turns the pointy-slots black.

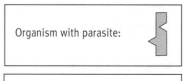

Organism with parasite:

Wait until the parasite invades the population quite severely. We end up with a nice mix of black and white pointy-slots.

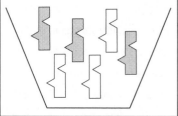

STEP 2 Add a mutation to the population's nuclear DNA designed to inhibit gametes from passing on some of their cytoplasmic elements. Mutations are common in all populations; they usually appear because of sunlight, pollution or some other agent. I'll refer to the mutation as 'cytoplasm-reducer' or CR. Now CR should be detrimental enough to the health of the population so that if two gametes that have it unite, they are doomed from a lack of healthy cytoplasm. In the pointy-slots' case the muta-tion cracks points and if two organisms with cracked points mate, offspring formation is doomed.

The upside is CR will help prevent the transmittal of parasites—in other words, the cracks will help prevent the black pointy-slots from having black offspring. So, you see, CR with

Organisms with CR mutation:

the parasite certainly makes for a good combination of ingredients.

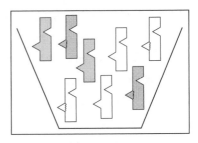

Wait until many organisms contain the CR mutation.

We end up with a population mix of: original organisms (white pointy-slots), original with parasite (black pointy-slots), original with mutation (cracked white pointy-slots), and original with parasite as well as mutation (cracked black pointy-slots).

STEP 3   Add another mutation to the population's nuclear DNA that prevents CR carriers from producing offspring with other CR carriers—this was a doomed event anyway. Organisms with this second mutation lose the freedom to have offspring with any other organism. For the pointy-slots, the mutation makes cracked points drop off and so any two 'point-less' organisms will not be able to reproduce. All other organisms, however, still enjoy the variety that comes with being able to reproduce with any other organism. We have the budding of a differentiation between sexes, so let's call this point-less mutation 'Sex 1'. Pointy-slots with Sex 1 can be white or black, with or with-out parasite, but they only have slots. What is important is that Sex 1 re-duces the unhealthy joining of two gametes both unable to donate all their cytoplasm—again, an ingre-dient that works well.

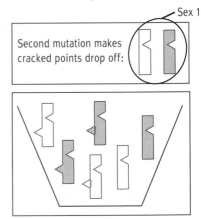

Second mutation makes cracked points drop off:

Sex 1

Wait until many organisms contain this second mutation.

STEP 4   Add a third mutation to the population's nuclear DNA, similar to the previous one, preventing its carrier from mating with other carriers. In our example, this makes slots become points. Now it doesn't matter how this mutation is added or which organisms cop it, if you wait long enough eventually it will become another sex—let's call this 'slot-less' mutation 'Sex 2'. At first some organisms could even contain both the Sex 1 and the Sex 2 mutation, but you should trust the recipe . . . with time things will separate out: organisms will only contain one or the other. So even if at some stage our population of pointy-slots includes organisms with all the possible mixes of the parasite and mutations, sooner or later everything will die down. And see how the pointy-slots end up? Double-pointed or single-slotted: only carrying the slot-less Sex 2 mutation or the point-less Sex 1 mutation. The recipe has worked. We have a division between two sexes, a bisexual population.

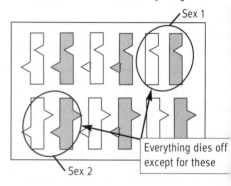

Sex 1

Everything dies off except for these

Sex 2

So according to this recipe, sexes emerge as mutations to fight off the original parasite. At this stage, I feel like going to the stove and saying: 'Here is one I prepared earlier' so you can see the end result, all beautifully prepared and presented. And like all cooking shows, everything seems simple enough. Especially when you think of the end result of this recipe. But there is a significant aspect of the preparation that's missing here. You can't just mash all these ingredients together as if you were making a mud pie. Creating sexuality is a more delicate and intricate procedure. But just how delicate and intricate is it? How do these ingredients combine? Is the creation of sexuality something to be expected, something easy to manufacture? Is the recipe easy or hard to follow? Can I let the pot simmer while I am watching TV in the other room, or do I have to continually monitor the situation carefully? You have to examine each step mathematically to reveal the finer details. Mathematics tells you exactly how each ingredient has to be measured and added to ensure the recipe is a success. Here is where the real work begins . . .

Step 1   Adding the parasite

For the initial parasite to invade the population, the organisms carrying it must proliferate. How detrimental can the parasite be without harming its host so much that it places its own successful survival in jeopardy? Well, this much:

$$w > (1 - p_E)/[2 - p_E(1 + \alpha)],\ 0.5 < w < 1,\ 0 < \alpha \leq 1.$$

You might have expected a concrete number, like the parasite holders have to be at least 80 per cent as fit as non-parasite holders. But then you would also have to quantify how fit parasite-free organisms are; how quickly the parasite spreads; the number of organisms resulting from the mating between two infected organisms and infected with a double dose of the parasite; and the relative fitness of organisms infected with such double doses. If someone were to try and specify all the possibilities that could arise from all these factors, they could come up with numbers rather than formulae. But they would also be faced with innumerable calculations and should be willing to never go out clubbing again in order to pursue the activity. Trust me, it's much easier to whack it all into an equation, and then go out and have a drink!

Step 2   Adding the cytoplasm-reducer (CR)

CR is the mutation that prevents its gamete carriers from transmitting elements of their cytoplasm. The recipe says: 'Wait until many organisms contain the mutation.' But can this actually happen? Or will I be waiting and waiting and waiting—and waiting? Mathematics says it can happen and in fact it tells you how many to expect:

$$0 < \hat{p}_A < 1, \ \hat{p}_A = \alpha / (1 + \alpha).$$

Again, no numbers until we find a volunteer willing to sacrifice their lives to perform innumerable, interminable detailed calculations. Calculations that have no real use either, since a mathematician looks at this equation and can see exactly what is happening anyway. As a mathematician you can see the pattern of how many to expect depending on the situation. In fact, numbers would only confuse things. Again, trust me: the equation is better.

Step 3   Adding Sex 1

Sex 1 is the mutation preventing CR carriers from joining with other CR carriers. This may sound like a sophisticated addition, but it doesn't have to be. All that is needed is something like a faulty chemical or receptor to develop, and in one clean swoop the whole gamete-joining process could be boycotted. OK, but if this were left to chance, what are the odds of this mutation appearing and then spreading thoroughly into the mix? To answer this question, you need what is called a matrix that looks like this:

$$gM = \begin{bmatrix} k_1 p_{00}^2 & k_1 p_{10} p_{00} & p_{01} p_{00} & p_{11} p_{00} \\ k_1 p_{00} p_{10} & k_1 p_{10}^2 & p_{01} p_{10} & p_{11} p_{10} \\ p_{00} p_{01} & p_{10} p_{01} & 0 & 0 \\ p_{00} p_{11} & p_{10} p_{11} & 0 & 0 \end{bmatrix}.$$

Unlike most people, whenever a mathematician hears 'the matrix', they get bombarded by images like the one above, not a leather-clad Keanu bouncing off walls. Yes, it's sad. But the trade-off is you get to understand theories like this one. Here the matrix helps you find out this second mutation requires some very delicate handling. Only in very rare cases will many organisms carry it. The more likely scenario is a gradual decline to its extinction.

Step 4   Adding Sex 2

Sex 2 is the mutation all organisms without the Sex 1 mutation end up with. It also prevents its gamete carriers from joining with other gamete carriers. More matrices show that after Sex 1 has become part of the population, the appearance and preservation of Sex 2 is quite straightforward. It is as if nature has a need to rectify a disequilibrium caused by having Sex 1 only. It doesn't even need justifying with possible advantages for its bearers. Mathematics shows its mere appearance easily causes a chain reaction leading to it flourishing into an intrinsic quality.

Parasite–Mutation–Mutation–Mutation: these are steps to dual sexuality. Our very early ancestors may very well have followed this dance, with mitochondria eventually evolving from that first parasite, and a few delicate moments occurring at the developmental stage of the second mutation Sex 1. Take your eyes off the stove at that point and everything could indeed go off the boil. Our two sexes should never be casually dismissed as some basic easy progression which has evolved to ensure a more successful survival. Sexuality is beautifully special, an exemplar of precision. We have, at the end of our efforts in the kitchen, a delicate and delicious soufflé on our hands rather than scrambled eggs.

So cytoplasmic parasitic genes can account for why two sexes evolved from none, yet a question still remains. Why are we plagued by species with two sexes and not three, four or more? Laurence Hurst from the University of Bath advocates cytoplasmic parasite gene theory is still the reason. His conclusion arises from an initial observation that suggests quite the opposite though. If bisexuality evolved as a way to coordinate a uniparental inheritance of cytoplasmic material, in order to prevent parasitic elements from taking hold, couldn't other sexualities do the same? Can't trisexual populations, for example, organise strict uniparental cytoplasmic inheritance just like bisexual ones?

Time to revisit the population of females, males and memales, where each sex may procreate with any other sex. But now we zoom in on each sex to consider how the inheritance of cytoplasmic elements is coordinated. Imagine that female mitochondria are always inherited, and memale mitochondria are never inherited. This boils down to uniparental cytoplasmic inheritance. Female mitochondria take over when confronted with male or memale mitochondria, and male mitochondria take over when confronted with memale mitochondria. Every eventuality is covered. Cytoplasmic inheritance is tightly organised to avoid parasites. So what could go wrong? Well a few things can, as suggested by eight equations, similar to the following:

$$pw' = \frac{[pw((pw + ps)(1 - U) + qw + rw + v) + ps(qw(1 - k) + rw + v)]}{\overline{W}}.$$

By analysing these equations developed by Laurence Hurst, you can foresee the future of the population as it deals with its continual crop of mutations. In particular, Laurence Hurst wondered if a weakening mutation that forced biparental cytoplasmic inheritance could develop in one of the sexes. Some simple sums show this can occur without too much trouble and then something intriguing can happen. The mutation can weaken the population enough so another mutation leading to a fourth sex can emerge. A fourth sex slightly different to the others as it would only be able to mate with one of the other three sexes (not all of them). And once it etches its way in, Hurst's calculations show it could easily disrupt the entire sexual set-up so all but two sexes get wiped out in the process. Again, two sexes emerge as a stable set of affairs. It's not a foolproof process, which explains why there are a couple of organisms with more than two sexes, but in many cases it appears a good way to go. To avoid cytoplasmic parasitic genes it works well to have more than one sex, and if the system is to be robust it is best to stop at two.

Never feel cheated because nature has given us little choice when it comes to finding a partner. With this theory, it seems if there were more to choose from, they would probably all be substandard mutants anyway. Another illustrative example of why it is better to shoot for quality instead of quantity.

One final phantasmagorical point. There is concern some of our latest techniques for assisted reproduction may compromise the strict coordination of mitochondria inheritance (St John 2002). One procedure involves adding another egg's cytoplasm to the one meant for development, to give the egg a bit of a developmental boost. And through this technique, babies have indeed been born carrying mitochondria from both the original egg and the cytoplasm donor egg (Brenner et al. 2000). As couples are turning to such fertility treatments more and more to start a family, I suggest we keep a close eye on things. Could this inheritance of extra mitochondria be the weakness that allows a third sex to develop? You know, I'm brought back to thinking about the relatively recent proliferation of boy bands. Now I am finding it more than a little suspicious. Heard of a group called 'Memales' yet?

$$\partial x \, / \, \partial x + \partial x \, / \, \partial x + \partial x \, / \, \partial x + \partial x \, / \, \partial x + \partial x \, / \, \partial x + \partial x \, / \, \partial x + \partial x \, / \, \partial x$$

Why are there only two sexes? Population dynamics or cytoplasmic parasitic genes? Talk about a simple question with a complicated answer. The mere definition of 'a sex' involves the fields of combinatorics and graph theory. And the two potential answers I gave go down the road of differential equations and matrices. Just what is happening to the field of biology? I studied biology at school. Wasn't it all about dissecting frogs, examining various kinds of leaves and memorising animal kingdom classifications? That is still part of it, but that part is getting smaller and smaller. Today biology is tackling questions with such a degree of sophistication that words alone are no longer enough to describe the findings. Biology is becoming as mathematical as physics and engineering. And biology and mathematics departments at universities around the world are fostering thinkers in this area at all levels. New courses, conferences, academic exchange programs—it's all happening.

The Human Genome Project surely comes to mind. Mathematics has been critical in deciphering the thirty to forty thousand genes the project has found encoded in our DNA. There are plenty of fascinating things to discuss in this arena but let me not divert from the topic of sex. Dealing with HIV has been a huge mathematical exercise: from understanding how it spreads across the population, to finding how individual cells become infected, to working on how a drug can interfere with its processes. At another biological level, literally, in fact, a true understanding of how the ovaries and testicles work only comes with mathematics, which I dedicate the next chapter to—so stay tuned.

Mathematical biology is blossoming far beyond the Human Genome Project, HIV and our gonads. Neurobiology: we know neurones fire, but which patterns lead to which result? Structural biology: proteins fold into various shapes to carry out their functions, but how do they know what shape to fold into and how do they do it so quickly? Marine biology: if we concentrate fishing on a particular species, what happens to the others, and what will be left in ten, fifty, a hundred, years time? The list goes on. Are you beginning to see mathematical patterns everywhere?

I know sometimes I sound like a parent watching their child's performance in the school play. No matter what happens, if mathematics is involved, I give it praise and the full glory. I surely haven't given enough praise to the field of computer science for example. The development of this field in the last half a century has been pivotal to all our discoveries in mathematical biology. But furthermore, mathematics itself has gained a tremendous amount by interacting with other disciplines. Many ground-breaking mathematical ideas have come from having the focus of a topic like biology. Biology can give mathematicians great insight into which step to take next. Classifications like biology, mathematics and physics are misleading. All these areas hugely benefit from each other. Our environment is a complex mix of all fields.

There are also unexpected side effects from cross-fertilisation among fields. For example, incorporating mathematics in biology has a huge influence on how research is conducted. The more mathematics, the more thinking goes on before scientists hit the labs with experiments. And this means less experimenting. Not only does this lead to less resources being used—both environmental and fiscal, but animal lives are saved too. Hardcore environmental and animal-rights activists might like to change some of the focus of their picketing and protesting. Instead of being anti this or anti that, there's the option of being pro-mathematics. Lobbying governments to increase mathematics funding to save animals. That makes sense to me. And focusing on something positive always gives a better impression. There's also the selling point that a cure for AIDS or cancer may pop out in the process.

How much prouder could mathematicians be? I urge you all to go out and picket for more mathematics. Meanwhile, I'd better get back to the topic of sex.

Chapter 8

HOW
OVARIES COUNT
AND
BALLS ADD UP

Here's a sexy thought. Our bodies are always involved in one kind of mathematical calculation or another. It is subconscious. It is inbuilt. I alluded to this in Chapter 3, when considering the subconscious mathematical techniques we might be using to find that special someone. It seemed likely we had developed a soul mate search pattern through evolution to help us get hitched adequately. From strategies we might use to solve a problem, to bilateral symmetry, to regular heartbeats, we are bursting with patterns on all levels and mathematics is in action, and our ovaries and testes, our 'balls', are by no means an exception.

How do ovaries count?

Ovaries are full of follicles each holding an immature egg. Girls are born with about 500 000 follicles on each ovary. And that's all the follicles or eggs they are ever going to have. By puberty there are about 83 000 follicles left on each ovary and by the time they're 35, about 30 000. On average, women have periods every 25 to 35 days and this corresponds with the release of an egg each time. Usually one ovary delivers one egg one month, the other the next egg, and so on—left, right, left, right . . . Now if a total of 940 000 follicles are lost in 35 years, where do they all go? Not all the follicles could have delivered eggs because a woman would have a maximum of 300 periods, or ovulations, in that time. The answer is: they just die. Follicles are constantly growing and maturing their eggs at random in both ovaries. But only one makes it to full maturity each month. The ovaries are full of follicles at different stages of development. Most, and this can happen at any stage, will stop developing and decay. Isn't that very wasteful of the body? Doesn't evolution suggest we are very tight with our resources and almost everything has a purpose or can be accounted for?

Here are some more ovarian arithmetical facts:

★ Mammals have remarkably constant litter sizes—in our case it's one (well, that's the standard).

★ If an ovary is removed, litter sizes are not cut in half but stay the same—a woman with one ovary can still expect a period once a month and not every second.

★ If a fully mature follicle is removed, another may stop dying to ensure litter constancy.

So among the randomly maturing and dying follicles, how does the body know the correct number of mature eggs for the litter size has been reached? A process by which one egg is chosen seems quite conceivable—choose the biggest. But what process could ensure a higher number for larger litters is always picked? How does the body organise a repetition of the egg-choosing process at such regular intervals? There is a lot of counting going on here but no accountant on site. Something smart seems to be happening.

The menstrual cycle is a symphony of hormonal activities. And in the late '80s and early '90s, H. Michael Lacker from the Department of Biomathematical Sciences at the Mount Sinai Medical School in New York, Ethan Akin from the Department of Mathematics at the City College in New York and Allon Percus from the Department of Physics at Harvard University discovered patterns within the symphony that begin to link all the follicle arithmetic together.

The symphony analogy works well. A whole bunch of hormones follow their own courses of action, respond to various cues, interact with each other, and the result is cohesive motion. Is there a conductor? More than one: both the ovaries and the brain influence the event.

As follicles grow on both ovaries they release a hormone called estradiol. The larger they are, the more of it they release. So in initial stages of development, they don't release much. The brain responds to low levels of estradiol by releasing follicle-stimulating hormone (FSH) and luteinising hormone (LH), two hormones that promote follicle growth. This is a cumulative effect. So when there aren't any large follicles making large amounts of estradiol, the brain encourages growth. Many follicles grow strong and release more and more estradiol, while others seem to randomly atrophy. The brain continues growth promotion until a medium level of estradiol is reached, whereby it brings its production of FSH and LH right back down. The smaller follicles can no longer maintain growth with these small amounts of growth hormones and many atrophy. But the larger follicles, which are more sensitive to FSH and LH, still respond to the minimal amounts and keep growing. Estradiol levels keep rising until another level of estradiol is reached whereby the brain releases a burst of mostly LH. This surge is the nail in the coffin, if you like. The biggest of the best follicles releases its egg. We have ovulation. Many follicles atrophy. Estradiol levels have by now plunged and while the body waits to see if the egg is fertilised and implanted in the uterus, random follicles begin to wake up and grow again. If fertilisation and implantation doesn't occur, there's menstruation and the brain is ready to give the newly awoken follicles a helping hand by releasing FSH and LH once more. The whole process begins again. It is called a feedback loop. The brain responds to what the ovaries do. The ovaries respond to what the brain does. There is no rest. It's a loop-the-loop process.

Now this is a simplified version of the full story. There are a few other hormones involved and the brain's release of FSH and LH is actually pulsatile—another pattern. But for our purposes we have enough. We see a well-built hormonal cyclical pattern, a lot of atrophied follicles, yet still not much counting. How is the counting happening? H. Michael Lacker and his colleagues found this hormonal cyclical pattern was way more than enough to account for it.

They used the following mathematical encapsulation of the above follicle growth hormonal pattern:

$$\frac{dx_i}{dt} = x_i \{ K - D(X - M_1 x_i)(X - M_2 x_i) \},$$

$$i = 1,\ldots,N \ , \ \frac{1}{M_1} + \frac{1}{M_2} < 1, \ X = \sum_{j=1}^{N} x_j \ .$$

This takes into account estradiol, FSH and LH levels, as well as the growth plan observed by each follicle. We know the follicles start to grow slowly and then receive a helping hand from brain hormones, but we don't know the precise growth plan they follow. We don't have the right equipment to work that out yet. So the mathematicians made an educated guess and also assumed each follicle followed the same one. Yet, as you are about to see, this did not prevent the extraction of some crucial findings.

As mathematicians work, they may intersperse their mathematical analysis with checkpoints. After a bout of mathematics, they stop and reinterpret the calculations physically. They make sure everything still makes sense and fits physical reality before they go on. The first checkpoint on the road to the mathematics of the ovary: the natural divide between spontaneous and induced ovulation.

We are spontaneous ovulators. We release an egg once a month whether we like it or not (unless we are on the Pill, pregnant, too young, too old, too stressed, too sick, too depressed, too hungry, too sporty ... eggs like a balanced lifestyle). But many animals, like cats or rabbits, are induced ovulators. They only release eggs if they are sexually stimulated. For them, the follicle-selection process is separate from the one that triggers the actual egg release. Their estradiol levels rise like ours but instead of just rising and rising, they steady out. The levels become high enough to make them receptive to male advances, but not high enough to cause eggs to be released. Only if nerve endings in the vagina are activated does the brain respond to make that happen. When doing the mathematics you reach a fork in the road representing these two distinct possibilities. Pleasing. And so continuing the mathematical analysis then leads to

$$\text{if } \lim_{\tau \to \infty} y_i = \frac{1}{\sqrt{M}}, \ \lim_{t \to T} x_i = \infty, \text{ and if } \lim_{\tau \to \infty} y_i = 0, \ \lim_{t \to T} x_i = 0$$

for spontaneous ovulators, and

$$\text{if } \lim_{\tau \to \infty} y_i = \frac{1}{\sqrt{M}}, \ \lim_{t \to \infty} x_i = \frac{X_\infty(M)}{M}, \text{ and if } \lim_{\tau \to \infty} y_i = 0, \ \lim_{t \to \infty} x_i = 0$$

for induced ovulators.

In other words, and this works for both the spontaneous and the induced case, it doesn't matter how many follicles start to mature at the beginning of the cycle, or what their initial level of maturity is, in the end only a constant number will reach full maturity. The others will atrophy. And this happens even if a bunch of follicles are suddenly removed mid-cycle. The hormonal symphony naturally causes the growing follicles to split into two groups: a small group of ovulating ones (which could, in fact, consist of just a single follicle) and a large group of disappearing ones.

We have an explanation not only for why litter sizes stay about constant, but also why they remain so, even if an entire ovary is removed. Now the mathematicians did have to make up the growth plan followed by the follicles and did assume every follicle followed the same one. The real plan could be completely different and even individually tailored for each follicle. But the point is you don't need fancy clocks to get the arithmetic going. The mathematics shows a simple feedback system can naturally initiate precise egg counting. The randomness within the ovaries can induce order. Mathematics somehow captures the fact that the whole is greater than the sum of its parts.

Because assuming every follicle grows in exactly the same way is probably a little unrealistic, the mathematicians did pursue an analysis of differing growth patterns. Adding this extra ingredient to the problem, however, takes it into uncharted mathematical territory. The mathematics needed to analyse this situation strictly has not yet been discovered. In these cases, mathematicians can turn to computer simulations for help with the analysis. This is more experimental but not without intellectual beauty or mathematics and still can be a very powerful way to reach checkpoints that confirm the original mathematical idea makes sense.

Lacker and his colleagues' computer simulations of follicle growth with slightly varying growth patterns reveal once again the ease with which the feedback system, based on randomly maturing follicles, allows order. Constant egg numbers are released at regular time intervals. It all works beautifully. The computer simulations even show that once the pool of inter-acting follicles has decreased substantially the system is more easily swayed into deviating from the norm. For example, the system can lose track of mature follicle numbers, or regular time intervals between ovulation might become not so regular. Both of these relaxations in the system have also been observed in real life. As women age, even though the number of identical twins caused by single ovulations remains constant, the number of fraternal twins or double ovulations has been shown to increase. Are the ovaries beginning to lose count? Furthermore, close to menopause, periods can be quite irregular. Are they losing track of time too?

Both these observations serve as other good checkpoints, and also suggest a theory. Maybe our large numbers of follicles are not due to superfluous and wasteful overproduction. Maybe we need such large numbers to be active as part of the feedback counting process. Without them, the system just wouldn't work so wonderfully. Most plants and animals release huge numbers of eggs, often in the millions, into the environment. But for warm-blooded vertebrates like us, more care is given to the reproductive process. Parental investment means we are better off with small numbers of offspring at any one time. Yet having all evolved from common ancestry, maybe our hormonal feedback mechanism developed as part of a clever add-on feature to keep the numbers down.

It appears then that ovaries all tucked away and hardly ever noticed are mathematical geniuses. But just as impressive are the mathematical achievements of their male counterparts.

Men's hormonal splurge

Women's hormonal patterns and the moods that go with them have been done to death, so let me speak of men's. Men are abounding with hormonal cycles. Cycles with hormones that, just like women's can have significant effects on moods. And cycling right up there with the best is testosterone, that hormone almost synonymous with masculinity. Men do have a lot of it. But it's not the amount that counts, it's more the major role it plays in the development of a number of typically male characteristics such as facial hair, sperm and the penis in the womb. About 95 per cent of men's testosterone is made in the testes. The rest is made in the adrenal glands, two glands sitting on top of the kidneys (where women make some of their testosterone too). An important characteristic of testosterone is that as it circulates in the blood it actually comes in two forms: free and bound. The names say it all because when free testosterone is 'hooked' onto a particular protein molecule it becomes bound testosterone. This is how it travels to sites within the body. Over 97 per cent of a man's total testosterone is bound and 'in transit'. Now we know both types of testosterone have different effects on the body, though we are not exactly sure what. Yet making the distinction is important. A guy could be exploding with bound testosterone but if he hasn't got enough free testosterone circulating in his body, he won't be functioning to his full potential. Which could mean having to deal with a number of annoyances ranging from sleep disorders, to depression, to erectile dysfunction.

Both forms of testosterone have daily, annual and also lifetime patterns. Research on the daily fluctuations of testosterone in particular has kept us seriously busy since the '70s. How come we are still working on what a particular hormone does in twenty-four hours? I mean, we've figured out so much since then. We've got mobile phones, stealth bombers, lip collagen—so what's the hold-up? Well, leaving men's individual variations aside, the task involves a complication. There is no apparatus like a testosterone-meter you can just stick into a guy's arm that will continuously filter blood for a few days and come up with a reading. What you have to do is draw regular blood samples (sometimes they do this every two-and-a-half minutes), which are then sent off to the lab to be analysed. The result will be a bunch of separate testosterone measurements or numbers you have to fit a pattern to—a mathematical exercise.

Thankfully, one pattern in daily testosterone levels is repeatedly obvious in the numbers coming out of most studies. For example, once again in 1996, Spanish clinicians José Valero-Politi and Xavier Fuentes-Arderiu found both bound and free testosterone fluctuate according to:

$$Y_t = M + A_1 \cos\left(\frac{2\pi}{1440}t + \varphi_1\right) + A_2 \cos\left(\frac{2\pi}{720}t + \varphi_2\right),$$

which means like this:

Testosterone levels peak in the morning and reach all-time daily lows in the evening, especially free testosterone. What time exactly? This study showed Spanish men experience their morning surge at around 10.30 a.m., which aligns with studies of French and Italian men. By comparison though, studies of American, Brazilian, and Chinese men have pinpointed the surge at around 8 a.m. What time is morning? I take it, it's lifestyle. The Spanish are especially renowned for being party lovers! Don't they regularly eat dinner at 11 p.m., go out dancing at the local *discoteca* until 6 a.m., and then catch up on sleep at lunchtime? I'm surprised their testosterone has time to drop at all.

The cultural time differences suggest testosterone appears to fluctuate for behavioural reasons. That it responds to sleeping and working habits. The exact reasons though are still being investigated. Is light a contributing factor? This has been ruled out as blind men's testosterone levels exhibit the same pattern (Jones 1997, p. 100). What about nocturnal bodily rhythms? An Israeli research team lead by Rafael Luboshitzky found a link between the occurrence of the first REM episode of the night and when testosterone begins to rise towards its morning peak. Could postural change play a role even? New Zealand researchers, R. Cooke, J. McIntosh and R. McIntosh at the University of Otago discovered evidence suggesting this may be part of the reason why free testosterone shows more extreme variation than the bound type. The large protein molecules testosterone binds to don't circulate around the body so easily if you're lying down. And if there aren't as many of those molecules hanging around, more testosterone will eventually roam free.

But there has to be more to the story. Especially since this is not the only daily variation observed. In between this daily peak and valley, there is a regular stream of smaller peaks and valleys. They are thought to come about because of the way in which testosterone is secreted in response to the brain's secretion of LH. LH is secreted in the form of a pulse and testosterone appears to be following in tow. The brain's LH pulse is an important part of the hormonal system and I'll come back to it in a second.

As for the exact timing of the mini testosterone peaks, these vary from study to study. Men show definite patterns but they seem highly tailored to the individual. To give you some idea, according to Johannes Veldhuis and his colleagues from the University of Virginia, in terms of total testosterone we're looking at about one peak every 112 minutes (close to one every two hours). Remember, this pattern was drawn out from numbers, here representing testosterone levels gathered every 10 minutes for 36 hours—we must thank *cluster analysis* for the finding, a relatively new statistical technique.

But there are more variations! On top of these daily ones, testosterone also appears to vary seasonally. In 1998 our Spanish team mentioned earlier used an equation, not too dissimilar to their one above, to encapsulate the yearly peaks and valleys. They found total testosterone levels surge around May and free testosterone levels surge around July. But another couple of studies both involving Italian men have uncovered different total testosterone surge times. One found a peak in February (Guagnano et al. 1985), the other in September (Bellastella et al. 1986). Looks like men develop their own individual cycle here too. Individual monthly cycles have been noted as well (Doering et al. 1975).

And as if this wasn't enough, there's also an age-related variation. With age those testosterone peaks and troughs lose their intensity. Research led by Thomas Mulligan from the McGuire Veterans Affairs Medical Center in Virginia found it is likely for those peaks to be cut down by half. This appears related to many older men's troubles, like osteoporosis, decreased muscle mass and loss of sexual interest.

And then among all these cycles, other testosterone peaks and troughs can be brought on by stress, exercise, seeing someone attractive or not eating enough meat. Are there any behavioural traits that can be pinned down to testosterone levels though? Well, yes, it appears testosterone is linked to quite a few. High levels of the hormone have been associated with increased sex drive, need for orgasm, competitiveness, irritability, aggression, assertiveness, mental alertness, self-confidence and being rambunctious. Are there some tumultuous forces here or what? And all this is cycling through men's bodies all day, every day, all year. But they're there to be embraced. First, if you want to seduce a guy, forget about dinner and a movie, go for a breakfast rendezvous when his testosterone will be soaring and he'll be receptive to advances. Second, always ask for favours around dinnertime when he'll be feeling calmer. And if the favour thing doesn't work first off, maybe try hooking into one of his smaller testosterone cycles: wait half an hour and ask again. He may have needed that little extra testosterone drop. And if that still doesn't work, you could wait a little while longer and ask again, but I'd try food. He may just be hungry. That's always a problem.

Focusing on testosterone though is being very restrictive and not appreciating the male body. Men's hormonal systems also involve gonadotropin-releasing hormone (GnRH), LH, FSH, estrogens like estradiol, progesterone, prolactin, oxytocin, and the list carries on. Some of these hormones, like testosterone and estradiol, are made in the testes. Others, like GnRH and LH, are made in the brain. And of particular importance to the reproductive system is the brain–ball feedback loop that underlies the production of GnRH, LH, and testosterone. It is similar to the one in women linking up ovarian estradiol levels with the brain. Here's how it works. A drop in testosterone signals the brain to make GnRH, which in turn signals the pituitary gland at the base of the brain to release LH. LH travels to the testes and signals them to make testosterone. So testosterone levels go up and GnRH and LH secretion comes back down. Until testosterone levels drop again. And the feedback system goes on. Monitoring men's bodies shows the brain's release of GnRH and in turn LH is pulsatile, like a heartbeat. Blup—the brain releases LH (about every one to two hours depending on the man). In response, blup—the testes release testosterone. The timing of the testosterone release is still a bit of a puzzle, confounded by men's individual characteristics and the fact that there's a time lag between LH and testosterone pulses. But now you can see more clearly why men's daily testosterone cycles are scattered with the mini peaks and valleys I mentioned earlier.

So testosterone might be thought of as the hormone that embodies the essence of what is manly, but it is nothing without its mate LH. LH is an important part of the equation. In some instances LH has successfully treated low libido, erectile dysfunction and infertility (Crenshaw 1997). But it only works when administered in its natural pulsatile fashion. All these patterns are quintessential. In 2000, Daniel Keenan and Johannes Veldhuis from the University of Virginia with Weimin Sun from the PathoGenesis Corporation in Seattle focused on understanding the mathematical pattern behind the GnRH–LH–testosterone or the brain–ball set-up. It came down to this:

$$\lambda(t) = H_{1,2}\left(\int_{(t-l_{1,2})\vee 0}^{(t-l_{1,1})\vee 0} X_{Te}(r)dr, \int_{(t-l_{2,2})\vee 0}^{(t-l_{2,1})\vee 0} X_G(r)dr \right),$$

$$p(s \mid T_G^{k-1}, \lambda(\cdot)) = \gamma \times \lambda(s)\left(\int_{T_G^{k-1}}^{s} \lambda(r)dr \right)^{\gamma-1} \exp^{-\left(\int_{T_G^{k-1}}^{s} \lambda(r)dr \right)^{\gamma}},$$

$$T_L^k = \left[\min_j\left\{ T_G^j \mid T_G^j \ge T_L^{k-1} + r_L \right\} \right] + \tau_L,$$

$$N_G(t) = \sum_{j=1}^{\infty} 1_{\left\{ T_G^j \le t \right\}}, \ N_L(t) = \sum_{j=1}^{\infty} 1_{\left\{ T_L^j \le t \right\}},$$

$$S_G(t) = H_3\left(\int_{(t-l_{3,2})\vee 0}^{(t-l_{3,1})\vee 0} X_{Te}(s)ds \right) + \xi_G(t),$$

$$S_{Te}(t) = H_4\left(\mu(t) \times \int_{(t-l_{4,2})\vee 0}^{(t-l_{4,1})\vee 0} X_L(s)ds \right) + \xi_{Te}(t),$$

$$S_L(t) = H_{5,6}\left(\sum_{j=0}^{N_L(t)} \int_{(T_L^j-l_{5,2})\vee 0}^{(T_L^j-l_{5,1})\vee 0} X_G(s)ds \times \Gamma(t - T_L^j), \int_{(t-l_{6,2})\vee 0}^{(t-l_{6,1})\vee 0} X_{Te}(s)ds \right) + \xi_L(t),$$

$$d\xi_i(t) = -\delta_i\xi_i(t) + \tau_i(S_i(t))dB_i(t), \ \xi_i(0) = 0, \ \delta_i > 0, \ i = Te, G, L,$$

$$A_G^j = \int_{T_G^{j-1}}^{T_G^j} S_G(t)dt, \ A_L^j = \int_{T_L^{j-1}}^{T_L^j} (1 - e^{-\eta(t-T_L^{j-1})})S_L(t)dt,$$

$$M_i^j = \Psi_i(T_i^{j-1}, T_i^j) \times M_i^{j-1} + A_i^j, \ i = G, L,$$

$$Z_G(t)dt = [\beta_G + M_G^{N_G(t)}\psi_G(t - T_G^{N_G(t)})]dt,$$

$$dX_G(t) = \left\{ -\alpha_G(X_G(t))X_G(t) + Z_G(t) \right\}dt + \sigma_G(X_G(t))dW_G(t),$$

$$Z_L(t)dt = [\beta_L + M_L^{N_L(t)}\psi_L(t - T_L^{N_L(t)}) + e^{-\eta(t-T_L^{N_L(t)})} + S_L(t)]dt\,,$$

$$dX_L(t) = \{-\alpha_L(X_L(t))X_L(t) + Z_L(t)\}dt + \sigma_L(X_L(t))dW_L(t)\,,$$

$$Z_{Te}(t)dt = [\beta_{Te} + S_{Te}(t)]dt\,,$$

$$dX_{Te}(t) = \{-\alpha_{Te}(X_{Te}(t))X_{Te}(t) + Z_{Te}(t)\}dt + \sigma_{Te}(X_{Te}(t))dW_{Te}(t).$$

Which just goes to show once again not to judge a book by its cover! If you've ever thought the balls and brain create a one-track mind, then see the beauty of it, because there's actually a lot going on beneath the surface to make that thought happen!

Mind you, the amount of detail in this system of equations is amazing. In summary they describe what the hormone concentration levels are in the blood at any given time and the rate at which hormones are being secreted. But to get these numbers, a whole array of processes underlying the feedback loop have been considered. The researchers have zoomed right into the cellular level: how long it takes cells to synthesise each hormone; how long they store hormones for, if at all, before releasing them into the blood stream; how the amount they release is influenced by the amount already present in the blood; how long it takes for one hormone to travel to a site where it is going to have an effect (that's brain–ball travel time, for example). All this is in the equations. But there's more. Taking a step back from the cellular level and looking at the system, the researchers considered: how long levels of hormones can be elevated for and the effect this has on the synthesis of other hormones; how long different hormones survive for in the blood system; how not all the blood gets pumped through every square inch of your body as it circulates. (Only a fraction of the blood and its hormones make it to the target tissues. I take it this depends on how much blood your balls can carry, or how big or small they are? This sounds like a problem of geometry to me!) Anyway, all these factors come into play to form numerous patterns. Patterns that are also influenced by the fact that all these processes operate in an imperfect setting. Each cell is not going to secrete exactly the same amount of hormone time and time again, or the same amount as its neighbour. So random variations from a standard secretion rate are going to happen. Furthermore, the variations are not static, but are likely to increase with age. All this is built into the equations.

It may seem a little overwhelming. But this is how sophisticated our knowledge is becoming. And this is the level of detail we need to come to grips with if we are ever going to understand how all our hormones interact exactly, and what their levels really are. We could work on building equipment like the testosterone-meter I spoke about before. But equations are better. It is highly unlikely that some hormone concentrations, like those of GnRH, will ever be able to be measured directly in humans. And with equations, you don't just get a reading of the continuous change in hormone levels: you also get a handle on the mechanisms driving them. What drives men's passions, desires and mood swings? Now the focus is on testing the mathematics to see if its predictions work, and fine-tuning and more testing where it doesn't. We're on to it.

$$\partial x / \partial x + \partial x / \partial x + \partial x / \partial x + \partial x / \partial x + \partial x / \partial x + \partial x / \partial x + \partial x / \partial x$$

Understanding the mathematical patterns of our hormonal systems has a great number of uses. H. Michael Lacker and his colleague's mathematics of the brain–ovaries hormonal system has since been used as a model from which to understand a common cause of infertility: polycystic ovary syndrome (Chávez-Ross et al. 1997). The mathematics has also been extended to refine artificial ovulating techniques in sheep and cattle (Soboleva et al. 2000). Testosterone replacement therapy has been significantly improved by making drug delivery follow the oscillations imposed by the body (Place & Nichols 1991). And the incredibly detailed mathematics of the brain–ball hormonal set-up is being used to identify reasons for why it begins to fail as men age (Keenan & Veldhuis 2001), not to mention giving us a glimpse into what lies ahead when it comes to future research on how our bodies work in general.

But I also find all this mathematics useful on a personal level. I feel sensitised to what life has on offer. Feedback loops, like those linking our brains with our gonads, are in action just about everywhere. Every time you eat, your blood sugar levels go up, your pancreas responds by releasing insulin, the insulin helps your cells absorb the sugar, your blood sugar level drops, and insulin production goes down. When bee colonies get hot, the bees fan their wings near the nest entrance to draw air in, the nest cools down, and the bees no longer fan. The economy too can be thought of as a feedback system. Consumer demand increases prices, increased prices lead to less demand, less demand leads to price decreases, and so on.

And then there's another pattern. Order out of randomness. The brain–ovaries model speaks of the possibility of regular ovulation in a system of randomly maturing follicles. Some research shows our brains also develop according to such a pattern. Neural connections in certain parts of our brain, like those in the frontal area, begin to develop randomly at birth and can have increased by 50 per cent by the time we are two. Once adolescence is over, however, neural connections have been reduced again and the brain seems unchanged from what it was at birth. This increase and decrease in connectivity in early years is necessary for proper brain functioning. The system seems to structure itself through this instigation of random connections (Edelman 1987; Bruer 1999). One of a mathematician's jobs is to search for such self-organising systems where order is likely to erupt from randomness.

Patterns, whether they're feedback loops, order out of randomness, or something else, are repeated across fields, and can be found on all scales. There are no boundaries in any direction. Are you starting to see why I love mathematics so much? Mathematics is a continual search for patterns. And life is a network of moving patterns. The more mathematics you do the more of these patterns you see. It sounds as if it could be confusing, but it isn't. It has a way of putting life into perspective. All the while remaining appreciative of its complexity. Of course, I would like to be able to take this further and say when I see a guy adjusting himself in public all I see is *stochastic differential equations* engendering *self-organisation*. Sorry, mathematics is good, but it's not that good!

Chapter 9

ORGASM

I always compare good exercise sessions to wild orgasmic sex. It's hard work, you're out of breath, there's sweat, sometimes cramps, but you stay driven and get into that zone that enables you to persevere to the end point, whereby you sit back, relaxed, all happy about your achievements. OK, I have been accused of being a gym junky. But what does it feel like then? Have you ever tried to describe it? Better still, have you ever wondered how your description of orgasm would match up with someone's of the opposite sex?

I guess on average women make more noise and fuss than men. But does this mean they are experiencing different sensations? Are women reaching higher levels of satisfaction? Can pleasure be rated according to vocal efforts and shudders?

How do male and female orgasms compare?

Back in 1976, Ellen Vance and Nathaniel Wagner working in the Department of Psychology at the University of Washington studied this very question. They first asked 300 students to describe their orgasmic experience and then asked 70 judges who had no knowledge of the sexes to 'sex-identify' 48 of them. Why only 48? They didn't want descriptions that were too brief as this might not be fair to the judges; they didn't want descriptions with bits that were clearly male or female, like 'my penis gets really hard'; and they didn't want descriptions with certain writing styles that may sway the identification (as men and women had been known to differ in their use of descriptive language in some studies). All this left them with 124 descriptions, of which they randomly selected 24 male ones and 24 female ones for the judges to classify.

Want to see a few?

'An orgasm feels like heaven in the heat of hell; a tremendous buildup within of pleasure that makes the tremendous work of releasing that pleasure worthwhile.'

'Begins with tensing and tingling in anticipation, rectal contractions starting series of chills up spine. Tingling and buzzing sensations grow suddenly to explosion in genital area, some sensation of dizzying and weakening—almost loss of conscious sensation, but not really. Explosion sort of flowers out to varying distance from genital area, depending on intensity.'

'A buildup of tension which starts to pulsate very fast, and then there is a sudden release from the tension and desire to sleep.'

Yes, mine would probably start something along the lines of: 'It is like getting those two extra reps out while doing chest press.'

So 48 descriptions like these were given to obstetrician-gynaecologists, clinical psychologists and medical students, for classification as male or female. The result? One medical student got 33 out of the 48 right, but the other 69 judges weren't successful at this task at all. The statistical analysis isn't riveting, so I'll leave it out, but the conclusion was: descriptions of orgasms are not sex distinguishable. First thing that comes to mind: Could a group that included Jack Nicholson, Gene Simmons from Kiss, and Madonna, have scored some '48 out of 48's? There is an assumption that obstetrician-gynaecologists, clinical psychologists, and medical students are orgasm experts, so while this study is not bad, it is far from conclusive. And then there was also that big cull of descriptions at the start. With all that interference, objectivity could have been lost from the problem. A lot of work left to be done. However this line of research lay more or less dormant until 2002, when Kenneth Mah and Yitzchak Binik, two researchers from Canada, decided to re-examine the issue. The field of statistics has grown a lot since the '70s. A combination of mathematics and computer technology has meant the tools for experimental design, method and analysis have changed so much there has been the equivalent of an industrial revolution in the area. Kenneth Mah and Yitzchak Binik certainly found themselves in a much better position to learn more on the subject.

In all the topics I've covered, I have more or less stayed clear from statistical analysis. I have been determined to keep away from any mathematics that might even remotely substantiate the opinion that mathematics is some form of number juggling. But now I find myself at a point where I wouldn't want to be seen as dismissing this part of mathematics either. And this is also the opportunity for me to show that what might appear as number games from the outside is actually an amazing intellectual experience. Could it be as good as orgasm? Well unless we have some model of what the orgasm experience feels like, we can't make a comparison! And that model is what Kenneth Mah and Yitzchak Binik hoped to develop. Their methodology—get nearly 900 people to rate words for their capacity to describe 'it'.

First, they had to choose which words they were going to use. Through a preliminary study, just under 100 people rated over 100 adjectives as possibilities. The range covered emotional and physical experiences, from pleasurable to painful ones. These appraisals drew out 60 plausible orgasmic adjectives. To give you a flavour, these included: satisfying, euphoric, unifying, spurting and swelling. Interestingly or maybe reassuringly, no 'painful' ones made it in.

Having isolated these 60 words, they began their study. A group consisting of 523 women and 365 men rated the words on a scale of 0 to 5 according to how well they fit the orgasmic feeling. They did this twice, once in the context of masturbation and once in the context of sex with a partner.

Here's where the brilliance of statistics comes in, because somehow some sense has to be made of all these ratings. That's 60 words rated by 888 people, twice. You might think of comparing the top five highest-scoring words for men and women. Their similarities and differences should reflect similarities and differences in the orgasmic feeling between the groups. But a lot more information has been gathered and there's more to the story. Understanding what orgasm feels like should also include what it doesn't really feel like. So low-scoring words should also be examined. In fact, all the words should be lined up to see how they fare in the male and female scoring. We're back to comparing the two ratings of the 60 words by the 888 people. Statistics can deal with this. With *principle component analysis* you can isolate the words that drive the assessments of the feeling from the sea of words and scores. They stick out. You can then isolate the ones that play a secondary role in the assessment, or, to stay with the driving analogy, the ones that are in the co-pilot seat. And then you can isolate the words in the co-co-pilot seat . . . well, you catch my drift. And on this goes. You can classify the words into groups according to their importance in accounting for the results.

According to Kenneth Mah and Yitzchak Binik's calculations, the most descriptive words for both men and women were: fulfilling, satisfying and pleasurable. I was hoping for a little more creativity. Now I wonder what it means that they all arose from the context of masturbation? Does being single have numerous advantages we haven't contemplated? We can't stop at this level. We have to look at all scores. The second most descriptive words all occurred in the context of sex with a partner. For men they were: loving, unifying and close. For women they were: pleasurable, satisfying and fulfilling. Yes, women clocked in the same words at both levels. You might be interested in seeing the third most descriptive words too. I think they have a slightly different flavour. For men they were: shuddering, quivering and trembling. For women they were: euphoric, elated and rapturous. And on this classification went.

Now there is a degree of subjectivity in this analysis. Through the calculations, Kenneth Mah and Yitzchak Binik have the power to shift the classification to some degree. It is like classifying colours. Some things are obviously blue, others green. But when it gets into the aquamarines, it gets a little tricky. But with *principle component analysis* you can quantify how much you've been involved. And having *Cronbach* α equal to 0.92 for the women's ratings, and *Cronbach* α equal to 0.90 for the men's, shows they pretty much kept their noses out of it.

But conclusions about what men and women feel during orgasm can't be drawn yet. The next step is to search for patterns within the classification. And calculating the following 'fit indices'

Two dimensional model	χ^2 / df	NNFI	CFI	IFI	GFI
Men	2.11	.80	.83	.81	.73
Women	2.43	.81	.84	.82	.76

shows there appears to be a clear distinction between two perceptions of the orgasmic feeling: the sensory ones like 'swelling' and 'spreading', and the cognitive or more psychological ones, like 'pleasurable' and 'loving'.

From here the words are further classified with these two perceptions in mind, and then the data may be interpreted with statistical measures. Are certain feelings related? Maybe if 'satisfaction' scores highly, 'quivering' always scores well too? If a word is always associated with another, you have to be careful about how much importance you give it. It could be redundant. Something else to measure is how the scores compared when people assessed words in the context of masturbation or in the context of sex with a partner. The data is gone through with a fine-tooth comb. And there's something else that has to be added to the analysis. We mustn't lose track of the fact that we are aiming to make generalisations about what it feels like to orgasm for all women and men in the world from a group of 888 people. You have to allow for some flexibility, but then not go crazy either. Feelings are subject to interpretation. The calculations take this all into account.

Now while Kenneth Mah and Yitzchak Binik were at it, they took the opportunity of checking whether age, religion, education, sexual orientation, relationship status, days since orgasm, and duration of orgasm, had anything to do with it. They even checked method used to reach orgasm with a partner: intercourse, oral stimulation, manual stimulation from other, manual stimulation from self etc. Nope. Nothing. It makes no difference. Orgasm feels the same no matter what—though I have read that older (but not geriatric) and more educated people have higher orgasm rates (Mah & Binik 2001).

And after all this, what were Kenneth Mah and Yitzchak Binik's final conclusions? Women and men seem to feel the same sensations. And when having sex with a partner, the orgasmic feeling rates higher on the emotional scale—a little check that what the study is isolating is not complete nonsense. Only one real difference emerged between male and female ratings and that was men's higher ratings for shooting sensations. Which as Kenneth Mah and Yitzchak Binik naturally point out presumably reflects ejaculation. What they question though is the relevance of that difference. Do men really feel the ejaculation part? Or are they getting confused with the visual imagery? Maybe the sensation is not too different from the flooding sensations women feel?

So much to learn! But another piece of the puzzle fits as to what on earth it feels like to orgasm. (Aside from 'good', that is.)

Now apart from good dinner party conversation, how else can this information help? Well until you have some kind of definition of what an orgasm feels like, you can't really assess whether someone has had one or not, or how far off from one they've been, or why they didn't get there. And how can sex therapy work if this initial assessment can't be made? If someone can't reach orgasm, is it because of sensory or cognitive issues? How do various medications affect these components? What role does happiness in a relationship play? Also, research so far has focused simply on whether there's orgasm or not. With proper orgasmic measurements a range of orgasmic experiences may be accounted for. Furthermore, we don't really understand the impact of certain surgeries like hysterectomies on orgasm. With these surgeries, people's sensations might be dampened without us even realising it because we don't know how to measure the sensations properly yet.

Kenneth Mah and Yitzchak Binik's study focused on the psychological experience. There is also the biological and physiological experience, where again what happens to men and women bears many similarities.

Both male and female orgasms involve similar pelvic-muscle contractions and the intensity of the contractions appears related to levels of the hormone oxytocin (Mah & Bink 2001; Carmichael et al. 1994). Increased blood pressure and heart rate can also be expected with orgasm of both sexes, as well as surges in the hormones noradrenaline and prolactin (Krüger et al. 1998; Exton et al. 1999). The role of these hormones is not clear, but the surge of prolactin can last for over an hour. The belief is that it helps in letting the brain know the event is over and it's time to relax. And if it was the '70s, maybe have a cigarette? Prolactin also surges after vomiting, but that's for a different book (Crenshaw 1997).

Men can have multiple orgasms, orgasms without ejaculating and ejaculations without orgasms (Hite 1981). Women can also ejaculate. Female ejaculation, not believed to simply be a release of urine, is thought to stem from glandular structures surrounding the urethra. These structures harbour similar characteristics to those of men's prostates. And there is speculation they may play a role in what has been identified as the G-spot (Mah & Bink 2001).

But while all this insight into the orgasmic experience seems appreciable, the area most definitely needs a lot of work. What is clear now though is our research has focused way too much on the psychological experience of the female orgasm and the ejaculatory experience of the male orgasm. Male and female orgasms appear to share many more similarities than differences. Now if this does make it into one of your dinner party conversations, can you try and get an answer for why women then tend to make so much more of a racket than men? This is bugging me even more now.

$$\partial x\,/\,\partial x + \partial x\,/\,\partial x + \partial x\,/\,\partial x + \partial x\,/\,\partial x + \partial x\,/\,\partial x + \partial x\,/\,\partial x + \partial x\,/\,\partial x$$

Have I changed your sex life forever? Is your brain going to be flooded with equations next time you look into that special someone's eyes whether unknown across a crowded room, over a romantic dinner, or among the throws of passion in bed? Maybe not, but you know there will be plenty of mathematical patterns in action.

Before I began writing this book, I knew mathematics and sex were related, but as I researched the numerous topics I must admit even I was astounded to find out just how much. Part of my life's focus has always been to expose the prevalence and liberating nature of mathematics. And the more I do, the more fuel gets added to the fire that drives me. Mathematics plays such a huge role in our lives but it seems to hardly get a mention. Hence the popular belief that mathematics is some form of bizarre, mostly useless number crunching, and that there is no new mathematics to be developed. I constantly challenge that view. Mathematics is pervasive. Mathematics is creative. Mathematics is a form of expression enabling us to grasp concepts we couldn't otherwise.

In Chapter 7, I compared myself to a proud parent, always praising mathematics no matter what. I am guilty. In many of our human endeavours, big or small, mathematics has been an invisible member of the team. The Human Genome Project is hailed as one of the biggest breakthroughs in human knowledge, but it wouldn't even be a glimmer in either of Francis Collins', Eric Lander's or Craig Venter's eye if it weren't for mathematics. I like bringing mathematics to the forefront for a change. Mathematics needs to be seen more often. I believe a significant number of people miss out on the amazing aspects of life that mathematics reveals, and this could be the simple reason why.

I want to live life to the fullest, experience as much of it as I can. That is why I exercise so much, go clubbing so much, and do mathematics so much. I want to feel it all! And part of that philosophy is to also feel what it feels like to contribute to life. Mathematics is my way of doing that, too. I could try writing music, politics, or building something, but for now at least I'll stick with mathematics. You see, while writing this book I stumbled on a great new mathematical venture. Out of all the topics I have come across, orgasm seems to be the one most desperate for more mathematical input. As we've seen, orgasm is a complex event incorporating many different aspects of the body. Equations are bound to uncover some of the underlying mechanisms driving the complex orgasmic interactions. So here goes, at the risk of making a reputation for myself as a complete sex-crazy mathematician, which if I did would be ground-breaking in itself, I have started working on some mathematics of orgasm with my colleague, Bruce Henry. I can see the headlines already:

THE REAL MATRIX—COMING SOONER!
BLACKBOARD ORGASMS WITH MATHEMATICIANS
A BEAUTIFUL GRIND

Looking forward to seeing the article?

FURTHER READING

Introduction

Chaudhuri, A. (2000). Stars in our eyes. *The Guardian*, 13 January.

Mitchell, V.-W. and Tate, E. (1998). Do consumers' star signs influence what they buy? *Marketing Intelligence & Planning*, 16 (4), 249–59.

Tyson, G.A. (1982). People who consult astrologers: A profile. *Pers. Indiv. Differ.*, 3 (2), 119–26.

1 Love, sweeeet love

Bartels, A. and Zeki, S. (2000). The neural basis of romantic love. *Neuroreport*, 11 (17), 3829–34.

Berscheid, E., Dion, K.K., Walster, E. and Walster, G.W. (1971). Physical attractiveness and dating choice: a test of the matching hypothesis. *J. Exp. Soc. Psychol.*, 7 (2), 173–89.

Fisher, H.E. (1992). *Anatomy of love*. New York: Norton.

Gragnani, A., Rinaldi, S. and Feichtinger, G. (1997). Cyclic dynamics in romantic relationships. *Int. J. Bifurcat. Chaos*, 7 (11), 2611–19.

Griffin, D. and Bartholomew, K. (1994). Models of the self and other: fundamental dimensions underlying measures of adult attachment. *J. Pers. Soc. Psychol.*, 67 (3), 430–45.

Hatfield, E. (1988). Passionate and companionate love. *The psychology of love* (pp. 191–217). New Haven, CT, US: Yale University Press.

Jones, F.J. (1995). *The structure of Petrarch's Canzoniere.* Cambridge, UK: Brewer.

Peele, S. (1988). Fools for love: The romantic ideal, psychological theory, and addictive love. *The psychology of love* (pp. 159–88). New Haven, CT, US: Yale University Press.

Rinaldi, S. (1998a). Laura and Petrarch: An intriguing case of cyclical love dynamics. *SIAM J. Appl. Math.*, 58 (4), 1205–21.

——(1998b). Love dynamics: the case of linear couples. *Appl. Math. Comput.*, 95 (2–3), 181–92.

Rinaldi, S. and Gragnani, A. (1998). Love dynamics between secure individuals: a modelling approach. *Nonlinear Dynamics, Psychology, and Life Sciences*, 2 (4), 283–301.

Shaver, P., Hazan, C. and Bradshaw, D. (1988). Love as attachment: The integration of three behavioural systems. *The psychology of love* (pp. 68–99). New Haven, CT, US: Yale University Press.

Simpson, J.A., Gangestad, S.W. and Lerma, M. (1990). Perception of physical attractiveness: mechanisms involved in the maintenance of romantic relationships. *J. Pers. Soc. Psychol.*, 59 (6), 1192–201.

Sternberg, R.J. (1988). Triangulating love. *The psychology of love* (pp. 119–38). New Haven, CT, US: Yale University Press.

Strogatz, S.H. (1994). *Nonlinear dynamics and chaos: with applications to physics, biology, chemistry and engineering.* Reading, Mass.: Addison-Wesley.

Zajonc, R.B., Adelmann, P.K., Murphy, S.T. and Niedenthal, P.M. (1987). Convergence in the physical appearance of spouses. *Motiv. Emotion*, 11 (4), 335–46.

2 Marriage and the happily ever after

Andelin, H.B. (1971). *Fascinating womanhood.* Santa Barbara, CA: Pacific Press.

Frey, B.S. and Eichenberger, R. (1996). Marriage paradoxes. *Ration. Soc.*, 8 (2), 187–206.

Gottman, J., Swanson, C. and Murray, J. (1999). The Mathematics of marital conflict: dynamic mathematical nonlinear modeling of newlywed marital interaction. *J. Fam. Psychol.*, 13 (1), 3–19.

Hendrix, H. (1990). *Getting the love you want: a guide for couples.* Melbourne: Schwartz & Wilkinson.

Kalai, A. and Kalai, E. (2001). Strategic polarisation. *J. Math. Psychol.*, 45, 656–63.

Kreider, R.M. and Fields, J.M. (2001). Number, timing, and duration of marriages and divorces: Fall 1996. *Current population reports.* US Census Bureau, Washington, DC, pp. 70–80.

Martin, J.D. (1970). Note on a mathematical 'theory' of coital frequency in marriage. *J. Sex Res.*, 6 (4), 326–31.

Rogers Gillmore, M., Gaylord, J., Hartway, J., Hoppe, M.J., Morrison, D.M., Leigh, B.C. and Rainey, D.T. (2001). Daily data collection of sexual and other health-related behaviors. *J. Sex Res.*, 38 (1), 35–42.

Wile, D.B. (1993). *Couples therapy: A nontraditional approach.* New York: Wiley Interscience.

3 Road testing the bed

Brown, N.R. and Sinclair, R.C. (1999). Estimating number of lifetime sexual partners: men and women do it differently. *J. Sex Res.*, 36 (3), 292–7.

Corbin, R.M. (1980). The secretary problem as a model of choice. *J. Math. Psychol.*, 21, 1–29.

Frank, A.Q. and Samuels, S.M. (1980). On an optimal stopping problem of Gusein-Zade. *Stoch. Proc. Appl.*, 10, 299–311.

Gigerenzer, G., Todd, P.M. and the ABC Research Group (1999). *Simple heuristics that make us smart.* New York, Oxford: Oxford University Press.

Gilbert, J.P. and Mosteller, F. (1966). Recognizing the maximum of a sequence. *J. Amer. Statist. Assoc.*, 61, 35–73.

Quine, M.P. and Law, J.S. (1996). Exact results for a secretary problem. *J. Appl. Probab.*, 33(3), 630–9.

Todd, P.M. (1997). Searching for the next best mate. *Simulating social phenomena* (pp. 419–36). Berlin: Springer-Verlag.

4 Dating services

Aggarwal, C.C. (2001). Re-designing distance functions and distance-based applications for high dimensional data. *SIGMOD Record*, 30 (1): 13–18.

Aggarwal, C.C., Hinneburg, A. and Keim, D.A. (2001). On the surprising behavior of distance metrics in high dimensional space. *Database Theory—ICDT 2001, Proceedings; Lecture Notes in Computer Science*, 420–34.

Bellman, R. (1961). *Adaptive control processes: a guided tour.* Princeton, N.J.: Princeton University Press.

Beyer, K., Goldstein, J., Ramakrishanan, R. and Shaft, U. (1999). When is 'nearest neighbor' meaningful? *Database Theory—ICDT 1999; Lecture Notes in Computer Science*, 217–35.

Bulcroft, R., Bulcroft, K., Bradley, K. and Simpson, C. (2000). The management and production of risk in romantic relationships: a postmodern paradox. *J. Fam. Hist.*, 25 (1), 63–92.

Hinneburg, A., Aggarwal, C., and Keim, D. (2000). What is the nearest neighbor in high dimensional spaces? *VLDB Conference Proceedings.* 506–15.

5 Pairing up

Caldarelli, G. and Capocci, A. (2001). Beauty and distance in the stable marriage problem. *Physica A,* 300 (1–2), 325–31.

Gale, D. and Shapley, L.S. (1962). College admissions and the stability of marriage. *Am. Math. Mon.,* 69 (1), 9–15.

Oméro, M.J., Dzierzawa, M., Marsili, M. and Zhang, Y.C. (1997), Scaling behavior in the stable marriage problem. *J. Physique I,* 7 (12), 1723–32.

6 Action reaction attraction

Burt, D.M. and Perrett, D.I. (1997). Perceptual asymmetries in judgements of facial attractiveness, age, gender, speech and expression. *Neuropsychologia*, 35 (5), 685–93.

Byrne, D. (1971). *The attraction paradigm.* New York: Academic Press.

——(1997). An overview (and underview) of research and theory within the attraction paradigm. *J. Pers. Soc. Relat.*, 14 (3), 417–31.

Byrne, D. and Nelson, D. (1965). Attraction as a linear function of proportion of positive reinforcements. *J. Pers. Soc. Psychol.*, 1 (6), 659–63.

Byrne, D. and Rhamey, R. (1965). Magnitude of positive and negative reinforcements as a determinant of attraction. *J. Pers. Soc. Psychol.*, 2 (6), 884–9.

Cann, A., Calhoun, L.G. and Banks, J.S. (1997). On the role of humor appreciation in interpersonal attraction: it's no joking matter. *Humor*, 10 (1), 77–89.

Duck, S. and Barnes, M.K. (1992). Disagreeing about agreement: reconciling differences about similarity. *Commun. Monogr.*, 59 (2), 199–208.

Freese, J. and Meland, S. (2002). Seven tenths incorrect: heterogeneity and change in the waist-to-hip ratios of *Playboy* centerfold models and Miss America pageant winners. *J. Sex Res.*, 39 (2), 133–8.

Grammer, K. and Thornhill, R. (1994). Human (*Homo sapiens*) facial attractiveness and sexual selection: the role of symmetry and averageness. *J. Comp. Psychol.*, 108 (3), 233–42.

Johnston, V.S. and Franklin, M. (1993). Is beauty in the eye of the beholder? *Ethol. Sociobiol.*, 14 (3), 183–99.

Kowner, R. (1996). Facial asymmetry and attractiveness judgement in developmental perspective. *J. Exp. Psychol.: Human Percep. Perform.*, 22 (3), 662–75.

Langlois, J.H., Kalakanis, L., Rubenstein, A.J., Larson, A., Hallam, M. and Smoot, M. (2000). Maxims or myths of beauty? A meta-analytic and theoretical review. *Psychol. Bull.*, 126 (3), 390–423.

Levinger, G. and Breedlove, J. (1966). Interpersonal attraction and agreement: a study of marriage partners. *J. Pers. Soc. Psychol.*, 3 (4), 367–72.

Michinov, E. and Michinov, N. (2001). The similarity hypothesis: a test of the moderating role of social comparison orientation. *Eur. J. Soc. Psychol.*, 31 (5), 549–55.

Nyikos, L., Balázs, L. and Schiller, R. (1994). Fractal analysis of artistic images: from cubism to fractalism. *Fractals*, 2 (1), 143–52.

Pearl, J. (2000). *Causality: Models, reasoning, and inference*. Cambridge: Cambridge University Press.

Rosenbaum, M.E. (1986). The repulsion hypothesis: on the nondevelopment of relationships. *J. Pers. Soc. Psychol.*, 51 (6), 1156–66.

Singh, D. (1993). Adaptive significance of female physical attractiveness: role of waist-to-hip ratio. *J. Pers. Soc. Psychol.*, 65 (2), 293–307.

Skinner, M. and Mullen, B. (1991). Facial asymmetry in emotional expression: a meta-analysis of research. *Brit. J. Soc. Psychol.*, 30, 113–24.

Spirtes, P., Glymour, C. and Scheines, R. (1993). *Causation, prediction, and search*. New York: Springer-Verlag.

Sunnafrank, M. (1992). On debunking the attitude similarity myth. *Commun. Monogr.*, 59 (2), 164–79.

Thornhill, R., Gangestad, S.W. and Comer, R. (1995). Human female orgasm and mate fluctuating asymmetry. *Anim. Behav.*, 50, 1601–15.

7 Pick a sex, any sex

Brenner, C.A., Barritt, J.A., Willadsen, S. and Cohen, J. (2000). Mitochondrial DNA heteroplasmy after human ooplasmic transplatation. *Fertil. Steril.*, 74(3), 573–8.

Bull, J.J. and Pease, C.M. (1989). Combinatorics and variety of mating-type systems. *Evolution*, 43 (3), 667–71.

Hurst, L.D. (1995). Selfish genetic elements and their role in evolution: the evolution of sex and some of what that entails. *Philos. T. Roy. Soc. B*, 349, 321–32.

——(1996). Why are there only two sexes? *P. Roy. Soc. Lond. B Bio.*, 263, 415–22.

Hutson, V. and Law, R. (1993). Four steps to two sexes. *P. Roy. Soc. Lond. B Bio*, 253, 43–51.

Iwasa, Y. and Sasaki, A. (1987). Evolution of the number of sexes. *Mathematical topics in population biology, morphogenesis and neurosciences (Kyoto, 1985)*. Lecture Notes in Biomath., 71, 144–53.

Iwasa, Y. and Sasaki, A. (1987). Evolution of the number of sexes. *Evolution*, 41 (1), 49–65.

St John, J.C. (2002). Ooplasm donation in humans. *Hum. Reprod.*, 17(8), 1954–8.

——(2002). The transmission of mitochondrial DNA following assisted reproduction techniques. *Theriogenology*, 57(1), 109–23.

Sutovsky, P., Moreno, R.D., Ramalho-Santos, J., Dominko, T., Simerly, C. and Schatten, G. (1999). Development: Ubiquitin tag for sperm mitochondria. *Nature*, 402 (6760), 371–2.

8 How ovaries count and balls add up

Bellastella, A., Crisuolo, T., Sinisi, A.A., Iorio, S., Sinisi, A.M., Rinaldi, A. and Faggiano, M. (1986). Circannual variations of plasma testosterone, luteinizing hormone, follicle-stimulating hormone and prolactin in Klinefelter's syndrome. *Neuroendocrinology*, 42, 153–7.

Bruer, J.T. (1999). Neural connections: Some you use, some you lose. *Phi Delta Kappan*, 81 (4), 264–77.

Chávez-Ross, A., Franks, S., Mason, H.D, Hardy, K. and Stark, J. (1997). Modelling the control of ovulation and polycystic ovary syndrome. *J. Math. Biol.*, 36 (1), 95–118.

Cooke, R.R., McIntosh, J.E.A. and McIntosh, R.P. (1993). Circadian variation in serum free and non-SHBG-bound testosterone in normal men: measurements, and simulation using mass action model. *Clin. Endocrinol.*, 39, 163–71.

Crenshaw, T.L. (1997). *The alchemy of love and lust: how our sex hormones influence our relationships.* New York: Pocket Books.

Doering, C.H., Kraemer, H.C., Brodie, H.K.H. and Hamburg, D.A. (1975). A cycle of plasma testosterone in the human male. *J. Clin. Endocr. Metab.*, 40 (3), 492–500.

Edelman, G.M. (1987). *Neural Darwinism.* New York: Basic Books.

Guagnano, M.T., Angelucci, E., Boni, R., Cervone, L. and Del Ponte, A. (1985). Circadian and circannual study of the hypophyseal–gonadal axis in healthy young males. *B. Soc. Ital. Biol. Sper.*, 61, 343–9.

Jones, R.E. (1997). *Human reproductive biology* (2nd edn). San Diego: Academic Press.

Keenan, D.M., Sun, W. and Veldhuis, J.D. (2000). A stochastic biomathematical model of the male reproductive hormone system. *SIAM J. Appl. Math.*, 61 (3), 934–65.

Keenan, D.M. and Veldhuis, J.D. (2001). Hypothesis testing of the aging male gonadal axis via a biomathematical construct. *Am. J. Physiol. Regulatory Integrative Comp. Physiol.*, 280 (6), R1755—R1771.

Lacker, H.M. and Akin, E. (1988). How do the ovaries count? *Math. Biosci.*, 90 (1–2), 305–32.

Lacker, H.M. and Percus, A. (1991). How do ovarian follicles interact? A many-body problem with unusual symmetry and symmetry-breaking properties. *J. Stat. Phys.*, 63 (5–6), 1133–61.

Luboshitzky, R., Zabari, Z., Shen-Orr, Z., Herer, P. and Lavie, P. (2001). Disruption of the nocturnal testosterone rhythm by sleep fragmentation in normal men. *J. Clin. Endocr. Metab.*, 86 (3), 1134–9.

Mulligan, T., Iranmanesh, A., Gheorghiu, S., Godschalk, M. and Veldhuis, J.D. (1995). Amplified nocturnal luteinizing hormone (LH) secretory burst frequency with selective attenuation of pulsatile (but not basal) testosterone secretion in healthy aged men: Possible Leydig cell desensitization to endogenous LH signaling—a clinical research center study. *J. Clin. Endocr. Metab.*, 80 (10), 3025–31.

Place, V.A. and Nichols, K.C. (1991). Transdermal delivery of testosterone with Testoderm to provide a normal circadian pattern of testosterone. *Ann. NY Acad. Sci.*, 618, 441–9.

Soboleva, T.K., Peterson, A.J., Pleasants, A.B., McNatty, K.P. and Rhodes, F.M. (2000). A model of follicular development and ovulation in sheep and cattle. *Anim. Reprod. Sci.*, 58 (1–2), 45–57.

Valero-Politi, J. and Fuentes-Arderiu, X. (1996). Daily rhythmic and non-rhythmic variations in follitropin, lutropin, testosterone, and sex-hormone-binding globulin in men. *Eur. J. Clin. Chem. Clin. Biochem.*, 34 (6), 455–62.

——(1998). Annual rhythmic variations of follitropin, lutropin, testosterone and sex-hormone-binding globulin in men. *Clin. Chim. Acta*, 271 (1), 57–71.

Veldhuis, J.D., King, J.C., Urban, R.J., Rogol, A.D., Evans, W.S., Kolp, L.A. and Johnson, M.L. (1987). Operating characteristics of the male hypothalamo-pituitary-gonadal axis: Pulsatile release of testosterone and follicle-stimulating hormone and their temporal coupling with luteinizing hormone. *J. Clin. Endocr. Metab.*, 65 (5), 929–41.

9 Orgasm

Carmichael, M.S., Warburton, V.L., Dixen, J. and Davidson, J.M. (1994). Relationships among cardiovascular, muscular, and oxytocin responses during human sexual activity. *Arch. Sex. Behav.*, 23 (1), 59–79.

Crenshaw, T.L (1997). *The alchemy of love and lust: how our sex hormones influence our relationships.* New York: Pocket Books.

Exton, M.S., Bindert, A., Krüger, T., Scheller, F., Hartmann, U. and Schedlowski, M. (1999). Cardiovascular and endocrine alterations after masturbation-induced orgasm in women. *Psychosom. Med.*, 61 (3), 280–9.

Hite, S. (1981). *The Hite report on male sexuality.* New York: Ballantine Books.

Krüger, T., Exton, M.S., Pawlak, C., von zur Mühlen, A., Hartmann, U. and Schedlowski, M. (1998). Neuroendocrine and cardiovascular response to sexual arousal and orgasm in men. *Psychoneuroendocrinology*, 23 (4), 401–411.

Mah, K. and Binik, Y.M. (2001). The nature of human orgasm: a critical review of major trends. *Clin. Psychol. Rev.*, 21 (6), 823–56.

——(2002). Do all orgasms feel alike? Evaluating a two-dimensional model of the orgasm experience across gender and sexual context. *J. Sex Res.*, 39 (2), 104–13.

Vance, E.B. and Wagner, N.N. (1976). Written descriptions of orgasm: a study of sex differences. *Arch. Sex. Behav.*, 5 (1), 87–98.